Other Harvard Medical School Books
published by Simon & Schuster

Harvard Medical School Family Health Guide
by the Harvard Medical School

Robert L. Barbieri, M.D.
Alice D. Domar, Ph.D.
Kevin R. Loughlin, M.D.

Six Steps to Increased Fertility

*An Integrated Medical
and Mind/Body Program
to Promote Conception*

A HARVARD MEDICAL SCHOOL BOOK

Simon & Schuster
New York London Toronto Sydney Singapore

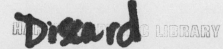

SIMON & SCHUSTER
Rockefeller Center
1230 Avenue of the Americas
New York, NY 10020

Written by Suzanne Wymelenberg

Illustrated by Harriet Greenfield

Designed by DEIRDRE C. AMTHOR

Manufactured in the United States of America

10   9   8   7   6   5   4   3   2   1

Library of Congress Cataloging-in-Publication Data
Barbieri, Robert L.
Six steps to increased fertility: an integrated medical and mind/body program
to promote conception / Robert L. Barbieri, Alice D. Domar, Kevin R. Loughlin.
p. cm
"A Harvard Medical School book."
Includes bibliographical references and index.
1. Infertility—Popular Works. I. Domar, Alice D. II. Loughlin, Kevin R.
RC889.B297 2000
616.6'9206—dc21   00-041335
ISBN 0-684-85522-4

Illustration credits appear on page 246.

This publication contains the opinions and ideas of its authors. It is intended to provide helpful and informative material on the subjects addressed in the publication. It is sold with the understanding that Harvard Medical School and the publisher are not engaged in rendering medical, health, psychological, or any other kind of personal professional services in the book. The reader should consult his or her medical, health, or other competent professional before adopting any of the suggestions in this book or drawing inferences from it.

Harvard Medical School and the publisher specifically disclaim all responsibility for any liability, loss, or risk, personal or otherwise, which is incurred as a consequence, directly or indirectly, of the use and application of any of the contents of this book.

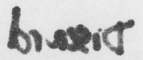

Acknowledgments

Warmest thanks to Sara DeLong for navigating the medical litera-ture with speed and an excellent sense of what was pertinent; to Marc O'Meara, R.D., for his expertise on commonsense nutrition for busy people; Barbara Nielsen, M.Div., for her guidance regard-ing the spiritual challenges many infertility patients face; and to all the women and men who agreed to be interviewed for this book about their experiences with infertility.

We also would like to thank our editor at Simon & Schuster, Roslyn Siegel, who believed in this book from its beginning; Anthony L. Komaroff, M.D., editor in chief of Harvard Health Publications, who brought us together and got us started, whose humor and enthusiasm were a great inspiration; Victoria Reeders, M.D., publications director of HHP, who is always ready to solve problems. And our immense thanks to our wonderful writer, Suzanne Wymelenberg, who not only was able to put our scien-tific articles and stray thoughts into lucid prose but also was so willing to track us down for answers to her questions.

To Sarah
(A.D.D.)

To Ronee, John, and Janet
(R.L.B.)

To my wife, Christine, for her love and support
(K.R.L.)

And to all our patients, from whom we've learned so much

Contents

Six Steps
to Increased
Fertility

Introduction

As doctors dealing with fertility problems, we see, listen to, and ultimately help hundreds of people to get pregnant each year. We know how concerned you become when another month passes and conception has not occurred. We know a great deal about your dreams and aspirations—and your frustrations and sense of failure. And we wanted to write this book to answer many of the questions and concerns we hear daily from you in our offices. Most of all, though, we wanted to write this book to reassure you that most of you will be able to conceive. Research has shown that although 20 percent of couples will be unable to achieve a pregnancy after a year of unprotected intercourse—the current definition of infertility—most of them will eventually achieve a successful pregnancy. Very few people have physical conditions that make it impossible to have a child, and in many cases, simple lifestyle changes and low-tech strategies can make a decisive difference. Besides, one year is far from a magic number—age and health differences and many other factors will influence your own chances of becoming pregnant.

If you do have difficulty getting pregnant, there is a great deal more you can do about it today than ever before. While assisted reproductive technology can help a large number of couples previously infertile, many couples can be helped by our greater knowledge of how lifestyle factors like stress, exercise, and nutrition affect conception, of better ways to regulate and target ovulation cycles, and of common medicines to avoid that can inhibit sperm and egg production. So much attention in the media is focused on the latest high-tech intervention that many people forget to give nature enough of a chance.

Each of us is an expert in a particular area affecting fertility. Dr. Barbieri, chairman of obstetrics and gynecology at Brigham and Women's Hospital, specializes in physical problems women have in getting pregnant. Dr. Loughlin, professor of surgery at Brigham and Women's Hospital, specializes in physical problems men have in conception. And Dr. Domar, the director of The Mind/Body Center for Women's Health at The Mind/Body Medical Institute, specializes in how the mind and emotions affect conception. We are delighted to be able to bring our separate viewpoints and expertise to this book. Like three pieces of a puzzle, we provide information that separately shows only part of the picture, but taken together creates a clear blueprint for success.

In this book we take a step approach to dealing with infertility. Just because we have sophisticated technology doesn't mean that everyone needs to make use of it. We believe that couples should always try the simplest, safest approach first before advancing to a more complicated and often more stressful and expensive intervention. In fact, for some of the steps in this book, you don't need a doctor at all.

Along the way you will meet a number of patients who have experiences similar to your own, and a host of tips and suggestions for maximizing your natural fertility.

But we will also tell you when it is time for the next step—the kind of tests and doctors that would be most helpful—and give you enough information to be sure you are getting the best available care. And because many couples are so anxious to get pregnant that they are tempted to skip important steps and jump to procedures that may not be necessary, we remind readers to always get a second opinion after a diagnosis and before starting a course of treatment.

One of the pleasures of this book is that you can start right now—today—without making a doctor's appointment, to improve your chances of conception. We hope this book can help bring you knowledge, peace of mind, and ultimately, a successful pregnancy.

STEP 1:
Begin Making Healthy Lifestyle Changes Today

If you are thinking about getting pregnant, you can do many simple, effective things right now to improve your chances of conception, because lifestyle can have profound effects on the reproductive functions of women and men. This means that increasing your fertility potential is something that you both can do without outside help: you can adopt healthy ways of eating, you can eliminate habits that may diminish fertility, and you can make sure your weight is within the range that's conducive to starting a pregnancy.

Think of this as a wellness program: Like an athlete, you'll be training for optimal performance. Not only can you enhance your prospects for a pregnancy, but as healthy parents you will be better prepared for the physical work of raising a child. Here are some simple strategies to pursue right now.

Keep Your Exercise Moderate

Women and Exercise

Getting enough exercise is an important part of helping your body to function well. But some women do so much exercise that it can be counterproductive, especially as far as fertility is concerned. A Harvard study by Dr. Rose E. Frisch examined the health of over 5300 women who had been athletes in college and found that strenuous or elite-level exercise appeared to impair fertility, which was often demonstrated by a lack of menstruation and ovulation. The most obvious indication that you are exercising too much if you want to become pregnant is having light or irregular periods or none at all. Professional or dedicated women athletes who want to have a baby need to cut back to much less strenuous levels of exercise or stop their workout programs altogether.

For the woman who already is experiencing infertility, Dr. Alice Domar and her colleagues at the Harvard Mind/Body Program for Infertility recommend that although giving up all exercise can be difficult for a woman who is concerned about weight gain or is used to exercising vigorously, she stop all exercise for three months to make sure exercise isn't a factor. Even when menstruation and ovulation appear normal, exercise can cause a decrease in progesterone levels that might prevent an embryo from implanting. Dr. Domar has seen a number of pregnancies result when women stopped exercising. Stretching routines, yoga, and relaxed strolls (under two miles) are good tension reducers and can be useful substitutes for vigorous exercise. A yoga program should be supervised by someone familiar with the effects of infertility treatments on the body.

Drs. Kevin Loughlin and Robert Barbieri, however, feel that a simple reduction in the number of miles women (and men) run or bicycle or in the hours they spend working out is sufficient to overcome most exercise-related fertility problems. Since exercise can affect body fat and a person's body mass index (BMI), its effect on fertility is difficult to sort out. For further information on the relationship between weight, exercise, and fertility, see pages 29–33.

LILLIAN'S STORY

In her job as a supervising chef at a well-known restaurant, Lillian was on her feet for eight to ten hours a day, with little opportunity to relax. "Our food had to be amazing, day after day, because we had a reputation to maintain. Something often goes wrong. It was exciting but demanding." In addition, Lillian ran for recreation and to keep fit. At five feet eight inches, she liked to keep her weight at 120 pounds. When she started attending the Mind/Body Program for Infertility, she had been trying to get pregnant for two years and the cause of her infertility couldn't be explained. She was thirty-three years old.

When she learned about the possible connection between too much exercise and infertility, Lillian slowed down. She gave up running and walked more slowly at work. As part of her effort to take life more easily, she also practiced the relaxation routines and meditation exercises taught in the program. "Overall, I became much calmer. For a month I gave up trying to get pregnant. I relaxed about everything, I didn't worry about when to have intercourse—and I got pregnant in six weeks. It was entirely unplanned." She now has a less demanding job and takes care of her baby.

Men and Exercise

Men can work out more than women without adversely affecting their fertility, but many research studies have found that high levels of exercise and endurance training can lead to a decrease in testosterone levels, negatively affecting libido and sperm health. Furthermore, men who are extremely lean can also experience marked drops in their testosterone levels, and may lose their interest in sex and their ability to have erections. Long-distance runners and scullers trying to keep to a lighter weight are examples of men who may experience infertility because of a combination of high-level exercise and lean bodies with little fat. These effects can be reversed with a modest weight gain.

We also should mention that over fifty miles a week of bicycling on a hard, narrow seat may lead to impotence. Studies have shown that sitting for long periods on such a seat can flatten the artery that controls blood flow to the penis. This type of bicycle seat may also cause nerve damage. Impotence specialists recommend switching from a solid seat to a type that has an oval opening built into the saddle. Various seats are available at bike stores.

Eat Well

An important influence on fertility is attaining a level of good nourishment that permits your body to function as it should. Bad eating habits can reduce the reserves of nutrients necessary for reproductive hormone systems to work properly. Inadequate nutrition also may weaken your immune system to the point where any sickness might diminish your fertility. This isn't just a woman's issue; men who don't get enough of certain vitamins and minerals may have low sperm counts and low testosterone levels.

It's important to eat regular, adequate meals—at least three a day—and to choose foods that are rich in nutrients and low in fat. And we recommend that you have one or two nourishing snacks every day as well. Good snacks help you avoid the temptation to reach for empty-calorie foods high in fat and sugar.

Eat More Fruits and Vegetables

This is the time to heed nutritionists' advice about stepping up the number and variety of fruits and vegetables you eat every day—currently the recommendation is five to eight servings per day. That may sound like a lot, but one serving can be as little as a couple tablespoons of raisins or a handful of fresh peas or grapes.

If you're not an enthusiastic vegetable/fruit eater and want to make each serving count the most, every week eat at least several dark green and orange/yellow vegetables such as Swiss chard, kale, sweet potatoes, and carrots, as well as red, orange, and yellow fruits. Deep-colored foods tend to have more nutrients. For instance, pink grapefruit has more nutritional value than white grapefruit, and watery-but-red watermelon is surprisingly nutritious.

GOOD HEALTH TIP

To make salads more nourishing, use lettuces such as romaine, Boston, or greenleaf (iceberg lettuce is not rich in vitamins) and include fresh spinach. Real time-savers are the lettuce mixes sold by most supermarkets. Because they contain a variety of greens, both flavor and vitamin content are better. For a change of pace that's quick, toss a leafy salad with a minimum of low-calorie dressing, and add several slices of ripe pear or mango to each serving. This looks elegant and tastes delicious.

A word about salad dressings: If you can wean your family from their favorite bottled dressings, it's cheaper and usually lower in fat and calories to mix a jar of your own. Do as Europeans do and toss the entire salad with just 1 or 2 tablespoons (or less) of dressing to barely coat the leaves so that the taste of the greens comes through.

Salad dressings taste better if they're made a day or two (or more) beforehand, well mixed, and stored in the refrigerator. Or mix your dressing right in the salad bowl as you start dinner preparations. Try crushing a garlic clove, then adding two parts olive oil, ¼ teaspoon of Dijon mustard, one part wine or cider vinegar or lemon juice, a drizzle of honey, and pepper to taste. Letting the dressing warm up to room temperature 30 to 60 minutes before tossing it with the greens enhances its flavor.

Although vegetables provide much of the vitamins, minerals, and fiber you need, if you are a vegetarian and are trying to improve your fertility, be sure that you're getting enough protein. Women who are vegetarians may have fertility problems because they have skewed levels of reproductive hormones: they metabolize estrogen into inactive products more quickly, and have longer menstrual cycles than women who include meat in their diets. Moreover, you are much more likely not to menstruate if you are both a runner and a vegetarian.

GOOD HEALTH TIP

One of the easiest ways to get enough fruit and vegetables is to use them as between-meal snacks. Supermarkets sell packages of baby carrots, cherry tomatoes, and assortments of bite-size pieces of melon that are easy to pack along to the office or to nibble on while watching TV. You can spend a few minutes cutting up broccoli and cauliflower or else buy a small vegetable party platter from your supermarket and use it for salads and snacks all week. (To wash away insecticides and other possible contaminants, thoroughly wash all precut vegetables and salad greens in water, add a few drops of dish detergent, then rinse well, before eating.)

To make a good accompaniment for fresh and cooked vegetables, add fresh dill, other herbs, or garlic powder to plain yogurt. And simply adding fresh spinach or slices of fruit to salads dramatically increases their nutritive value.

Snacks Can Be Good for You

Don't be afraid to eat snacks between meals. Choose snacks that are low in fat and salt, taste good, and make you feel satisfied, so that you can override any yearnings for high-sugar, high-fat foods. Keep several on hand for those times when your energy is flagging or you have the greatest cravings for junk food. See the box that follows for ideas for between-meals foods.

To make a snack more satisfying, combine carbohydrate foods with protein foods (see chart, page 26). If you don't want to gain weight, check the portion size and calorie amount listed on the food label to help you determine how big a snack to eat.

Snacks are also more satisfying if you eat them slowly and mindfully. Be aware of how much you're eating, how full you feel, and how it tastes. Avoid eating while you're doing something else to lessen the risk of thoughtless munching. Serve yourself one portion and put the rest of the food away. When you're very hungry and preparing a meal, nibble on chunks of raw vegetables such as sweet red or green peppers, cucumbers, or celery instead of reaching for potato chips. A more nutritious substitute for chips are whole-grain crackers such as Wasa Crispbreads, Kavli, Finn Crisp, whole wheat matzos, and Whole Foods Baked Woven Wheats.

GOOD SNACK COMBINATIONS

PROTEIN	CARBOHYDRATE
Cottage cheese*	Fruit/crackers/celery
Natural peanut butter (1 tb.)*	Bread/crackers/celery
Skim or 1% milk	Cereal (with less than 1 tsp. sugar per serving)
Low-fat/fat-free yogurt	Fruit/Grape-nuts
Baked tofu*	Crackers/rice cakes
Low-fat mozzarella cheese	Melted over tomatoes on bagel or English muffin
Bean dips/hummus	Baked tortilla chips/crackers/raw vegetables
Cottage cheese with herbs	Baked potato/bagel chips
Low-fat vegetable dips	Raw vegetables/crackers
Skim or 1% milk	Popcorn (air-popped)
Goat or low-fat cheddar cheese	Whole wheat crackers
Light or fat-free cream cheese	Bagel chips/crackers
Nuts (¼ cup or less)*	Dried fruit (2 tb.)
Tofu salad*	Bread/rice cakes

*Foods high in unsaturated fat

Food Supplements Help

In addition to eating a fruit- and vegetable-rich diet, both men and women should take a multivitamin/mineral supplement. Taking a single multivitamin/mineral tablet avoids the danger of taking too much of one vitamin or mineral. Megadoses of vitamins should be avoided, especially if they're fat soluble. Fat-soluble vitamins, such as vitamin A or vitamin D, are not readily excreted and can build up to toxic levels in your body, a particular concern if you're trying to get pregnant. This doesn't mean you should avoid these important vitamins, but just be sure not to take doses that are over the federal recommended daily allowance (RDA) without the advice of a nutritionist or doctor. RDAs are listed on the labels of vitamin bottles.

WARNING: LIMIT YOUR VITAMIN A

At any time it's wise not to take too much vitamin A, but this is especially important when you are expecting to have a child. A study of 22,000 women showed an apparent increase in the number of birth defects when pregnant women took over 10,000 international units (IU) of this vitamin. To be on the safe side, nutritionists recommend you choose a multivitamin that contains only 5000 IU of this vitamin. This allows you to also eat a lot of foods every day that are rich in this vitamin and in beta carotene, its precursor.

FOLIC ACID. A woman hoping to get pregnant should take a daily supplement that includes at least 400 micrograms (mcg) of folic acid. Folic acid is a synthetic form of folate (one of the B vitamins), and is now available in most multivitamin/mineral tablets and as a supplement in a few food products. Folic acid helps prevent anencephaly and spina bifida, birth defects of the brain and spinal cord, respectively. It's vital to have enough of this vitamin in your body *before* you conceive as well as afterward because such defects can occur within the first thirty days after the egg is fertilized. (It's also important, however, not to take more than 1000 mcg of folic acid unless your doctor or other health care provider clearly advises it.) Although you can get folate from foods, it is only half as available to the body as folic acid. The simplest approach may be to get the recommended minimum of 400 mcg every day in a multivitamin and think of the folate in foods as a bonus.

CALCIUM. During their reproductive years (and afterward) women also should consume about 1200 milligrams (mg) of calcium every day. To get that much, you will need to eat or drink at least three 8-ounce servings of dairy products, such as low-fat or nonfat yogurt and milk, or healthy fortified foods such as calcium-fortified orange juice. Read the product labels—they list serving size and the amount of calcium per serving.

If you can't eat enough calcium-rich food every day, a good way to make sure you're getting enough of this important bone preserver is to take a supplement. Calcium carbonate, calcium lactate, calcium citrate, or calcium citrate malate all are good, readily digested supplements. They are best absorbed when taken with a meal in doses of 500 mg or less. If you can't take your supplement with meals, calcium citrate is the form most easily digested on its own. Check the labels to make sure the form you buy is low in lead. Calcium derived from bonemeal or oyster shells can contain higher levels of lead. At all ages, everyone, male and female, should consume at least 1000 mg of calcium every day.

ZINC. Men, too, may benefit from taking a daily multivitamin supplement, particularly one that contains the RDA of zinc, which some researchers found is associated with the production of healthy sperm. An adequate level of zinc in the body is needed for the testicles to function normally. A deficiency in this important mineral also may decrease libido and contribute to impotence, probably by reducing testosterone levels. Other studies have found that a lack of zinc can reduce sperm count; however, the benefit of oral zinc on male infertility is still uncertain.

Increase Your Body Fat

For a change, this is not a suggestion to lose weight, unless you are very overweight. Like too much exercise, being too thin can delay puberty or slow down or stop menstrual periods entirely. To be able to reproduce, you must store a minimum amount of body fat. Teenagers need to have a certain amount of body fat in order to start having periods. A decrease in body fat can cause menstruation to stop. Women whose body mass index is below 17 are more likely to find that their periods have become further apart, are light, or have stopped, compared to women of normal weight for their height.

Body mass index describes body weight relative to height and is strongly correlated with total body fat content in adults. Its numbers apply to both men and women. The normal body mass index for adults is between 20 and 27. A six-foot-tall person who weighs 221 pounds or a person who is five feet six inches and weighs 186 pounds will each have a BMI of 30—and both would be considered excessively heavy. The new BMI guidelines, as developed by an expert panel, define overweight as a BMI of 27 to 29.9 and obesity as a BMI of 30 or more.

You can calculate your own BMI by multiplying your weight in pounds by 703 and dividing that amount by your height in inches squared. (For example, the square of 68 inches tall is 68 × 68, or 4624 inches.) If your weight is 150 pounds. and you multiply that by 703 you'll get 105,450. Dividing 4624 into 105,450 reveals a body mass index of 22.8—well within the normal adult range. See the BMI chart on page 30.

What's Your Body Mass Index (BMI)?

Your BMI is your weight in pounds multiplied by 703 and then divided by your height in inches squared. See below.

BMI	19	20	21	22	23	24	25	26	27	28	29	30	35	40
							Weight (*pounds*)							
Height														
4'10"	91	96	100	105	110	115	119	124	129	134	138	143	167	191
4'11"	94	99	104	109	114	119	124	128	133	138	143	148	173	198
5'0"	97	102	107	112	118	123	128	133	138	143	148	153	179	204
5'1"	100	106	111	116	122	127	132	137	143	148	153	158	185	211
5'2"	104	109	115	120	126	131	136	142	147	153	158	164	191	218
5'3"	107	113	118	124	130	135	141	146	152	158	163	169	197	225
5'4"	110	116	122	128	134	140	145	151	157	163	169	174	204	232
5'5"	114	120	126	132	138	144	150	156	162	168	174	180	210	240
5'6"	118	124	130	136	142	148	155	161	167	173	179	186	216	247
5'7"	121	127	134	140	146	153	159	166	172	178	185	191	223	255
5'8"	125	131	138	144	151	158	164	171	177	184	190	197	230	262
5'9"	128	135	142	149	155	162	169	176	182	189	196	203	236	270
5'10"	132	139	146	153	160	167	174	181	188	195	202	207	243	278
5'11"	136	143	150	157	165	172	179	186	193	200	208	215	250	286
6'0"	140	147	154	162	169	177	184	191	199	206	213	221	258	294
6'1"	144	151	159	166	174	182	189	197	204	212	219	227	265	302
6'2"	148	155	163	171	179	186	194	202	210	218	225	233	272	311
6'3"	152	160	168	176	184	192	200	208	216	224	232	240	279	319
6'4"	156	164	172	180	189	197	205	213	221	230	238	246	287	328

Overweight   Obese

Adapted from the *Nutrition Action Healthletter* and the World Health Organization.

The hypothalamus, which governs reproduction in both women and men, receives information from other sensors located in the brain. External factors such as stress, temperature, nutrition, and physical effort influence the hypothalamus. A combination of intense exercise and little body fat affects women and men much the same way: the hypothalamus secretes too little gonadotropin-releasing hormone (GnRH) or releases it in an abnormal pattern, which in turn affects the timely secretion of other reproductive hormones that are important to normal fertility in either sex. Produced in the hypothalamus, GnRH controls the production and secretion of follicle-stimulating hormone (FSH) and luteinizing hormone (LH), which in turn stimulate the ovaries and testicles.

In our female ancestors, this action of the hypothalamus probably evolved to ensure that conception would occur only when the woman's body had enough fat calories stored to nourish a fetus and then allow ample breast-feeding. Women who became pregnant when they were thin probably lost their babies or didn't survive themselves. This may have been the process of natural selection that led to the fact that women today carry more fat than men—about one-fourth of female weight normally is in fat.

BODY MASS INDEX AND FEMALE FERTILITY

BMI	*Relative Female Fertility*
less than 17	significantly reduced fertility
17 to 20	slight reduction in fertility
20 to 27	normal fertility
27 to 30	slight reduction in fertility
over 30	significantly reduced fertility

Excessively thin women have difficulty reproducing. We can see the effect of too little body fat today in women athletes who don't ovulate or who ovulate but can't get pregnant, even though their body mass index may be in the normal range. That's because most of their body is made up of muscle and, despite having a normal BMI, they don't have enough fat. Men's bodies, too, need some fat for them to maintain normal testosterone levels and healthy sperm. Body weight doesn't always reflect the amount of fat a body contains.

In addition, having a lower than normal BMI, even without strenuous exercise, may cause ovulation to stop "silently"—menstruation may continue and may seem normal, but ovulation doesn't occur. According to Harvard scientist Rose E. Frisch, the infertility that could result from this can be reversed by weight gain or less exercise, or both. Furthermore, a very restrictive diet can lead to low levels of progesterone, slow the growth of egg follicles (the fluid-filled pockets in which eggs grow), and inhibit the surge of luteinizing hormone (LH) that facilitates ovulation.

More recently, researchers have found that very thin women who gain weight and increase their body fat in order to conceive need to wait until their BMI is in the normal range before they try to get pregnant. Women who are on the low end of the BMI normal range may have difficulty in maintaining a pregnancy. Women need sufficient fat reserves to nurture a fetus.

Men whose BMI is 18 or less also may have reduced fertility. They are likely to experience a loss of libido and have decreased amounts of the prostate fluids that carry the sperm out of the penis and protect them after ejaculation. In addition, their sperm will be less active and shorter-lived. As in women, weight gain restores these losses.

Reduce Your Body Fat

The other extreme—having too much body fat—in women, at least, is also associated with long periods between menstruation (thirty-five days or more), a lack of menstruation, and infertility.

An overweight body produces higher than normal levels of certain hormones that then inhibit ovulation. The pregnancy rate for overweight women—women who have a body mass index that's higher than 27—often is reduced. (See the chart that compares levels of fertility with BMI levels, page 31.)

Exactly what hormonal changes take place when women have too much body fat is not entirely known, but researchers have seen that hormone levels return to normal and menstrual cycles become more normal when overweight women lose even as few as fifteen pounds. It appears that many women must be within a certain BMI range to have normal ovulatory cycles. Just as gaining weight can restore ovulation if you're too thin, losing weight can be very effective if the cause of your ovulation problem is overweight.

Drinking: Women Should Stop; Men Should Be Moderate

The effects of drinking beer, wine, or liquor on pregnancy have been studied for many years, but until recently there was little information available on the specific effects of moderate or no alcohol intake on reproductive capability. Studying more than 1000 infertility patients and 3800 women who recently gave birth, Harvard researchers in 1994 found that women who were "moderate" drinkers—who usually had one drink a day—experienced a slightly greater rate of ovulatory infertility. This risk was greater in women who had more than one drink a day. Endometriosis, however, in which fragments of the lining of the uterus are found in other parts of the pelvic cavity, was more common in women who drank, regardless of the amount. Both of these problems are linked to hormone function, which appears to be affected by alcohol intake.

Furthermore, in 1998, two studies emphasized the negative effects of alcohol on fertility: In a Danish study of 430 couples, women who drank moderately (fewer than five drinks a week) reduced their chances of conception, compared to women who didn't drink alcohol at all. *In fact, the ability to become pregnant decreased steadily in a direct relationship to the amount of alcohol intake. Among women who had more than ten drinks a week, the odds of getting pregnant were about half those of the women who had fewer than five per week.* The couples studied were between the ages of twenty and thirty-five and were trying to conceive for the first time. Among the male partners no association was found between alcohol intake and the couple's rate of conception. Most of the women in this study drank wine.

Research at Johns Hopkins University reinforced the Danish findings: Women who avoided both alcohol and caffeine were more than two and a half times as likely to conceive as women who consumed any alcohol and drank more than one cup of coffee a day. The highest conception rate was among women who didn't drink, didn't smoke, and had less than a cup of coffee or its equivalent per day.

Alcohol and Miscarriage

Alcohol also can endanger a pregnancy. According to some studies, the risk of spontaneous abortion (miscarriage) appears to increase with moderate drinking during the early weeks of pregnancy, particularly the first ten weeks. If a woman has one drink a day during the first trimester of pregnancy, her risk of a spontaneous abortion is about double that of the woman who doesn't drink at all. Other research, however, particularly in Europe, has not confirmed this association, so more studies are needed to resolve the issue.

In addition to the possibility that moderate alcohol intake may lead to ovulatory infertility or to a miscarriage, two or three bottles of beer or glasses of wine or two mixed drinks per day can have a detrimental effect on fetal development. Babies may be born with fetal alcohol syndrome, a combination of birth defects that result from this level of alcohol consumption by the mother during pregnancy. An embryo can be affected by any toxins in its mother's system, especially during the first two to six weeks of its development, a time when many women don't realize they are pregnant. And a chronic high blood-alcohol level during the third trimester may cause a growth deficiency and contribute to mental retardation in the infant. Practically speaking, there is no safe level of alcohol intake during pregnancy.

In men, some studies have found a link between heavy drinking and a reduction in testicle size, infertility, and/or decreased libido and impotence. Although the Danish study we mentioned shows no relationship between drinking alcohol and male fertility, other researchers have found that alcohol consumption produces significant changes in the shape of sperm and their ability to move. Furthermore, in men who are chronically heavy drinkers, the sperm production structure of the testicles becomes damaged so fewer mature sperm develop. Research shows that having more than one drink a day can interfere with testosterone secretion, reducing a man's sex drive and ability to produce mature sperm.

If you want to enhance your chances of conceiving, the bottom line seems to be that women should give up alcohol, coffee, and cigarettes and men should moderate their use of these stimulants.

Decrease Your Caffeine Consumption

Since 1988 there have been numerous studies regarding the effects of caffeine on a woman's fertility. Although the results are not totally definitive, there is enough information to recommend that you be cautious in your caffeine intake. A 1997 report on more than 3000 women in five European countries said that women who drank more than five cups (500 mg) of brewed coffee a day experienced delays in conceiving. This delay was increased if the woman was a smoker. The Johns Hopkins research on alcohol and caffeine consumption shows that more than a single cup of coffee a day can have a negative effect on fertility. And an earlier U.S. study found that a woman's chances of becoming pregnant were reduced if she drank more than three cups (300 mg) of brewed coffee daily. Furthermore, the combination of smoking and coffee drinking was associated with a significantly increased risk of delayed conception. We should point out that most coffee today is sold in 8-ounce cups that, on the average, hold 135 mg of caffeine, which is more than the 100 mg cups the studies describe. Three cups of takeout coffee will equal 405 mg of caffeine.

Caffeine also may be linked to a higher-than-normal risk of miscarriage, but the jury still seems to be out on this issue. A recent large study in Connecticut found a strong link between caffeine consumption and spontaneous abortion, while an even larger study in California found no such association.

Figure Out Your Caffeine Intake

If you want to estimate your caffeine intake, measure what your mug or cup holds. A full 8-ounce cup of most brewed coffees has approximately 135 mg of caffeine, a cup of instant coffee has 65 mg, a cup of tea 50 mg, 12 ounces of a soft drink contain 60 mg, and 12 ounces of a *diet* soft drink provide 78 mg of caffeine. Decaffeinated coffee has only 2 mg per 8 ounces. Cups of coffee offered at some coffeehouses may supply more than 135 mg of caffeine, however. The amount can vary from one establishment to another and from one type of coffee to another.

Some over-the-counter drug products also contain significant amounts of caffeine. These include NoDoz, a product designed to help people stay awake, and the headache painkillers Excedrin and Anacin. One tablet of Maximum Strength NoDoz provides 200 mg and one tablet of Regular Strength has 100 mg of caffeine. Two tablets of Excedrin add up to 130 mg of caffeine and two tablets of Anacin together have 65 mg.

Even though the question of the effect of caffeine on the length of time it takes to conceive is not entirely settled, you may want to enhance your chances by switching to decaffeinated coffee or tea. If you're a serious coffee drinker, reduce your consumption very slowly—by a half cup per week—to avoid withdrawal problems such as headaches or fatigue.

Give Up Nicotine, Marijuana, Cocaine, and Steroids

Tobacco smoking has been linked to reduced fertility in both women and men. In addition, a recent British study has found an association between smoking and stillbirths, low birthweight babies, and sudden infant death syndrome (SIDS). A woman who smokes is likely to have less chance of becoming pregnant and giving birth when treated with in vitro fertilization (IVF) than a woman who doesn't smoke. This is especially true if she smokes twenty or more cigarettes a day. A mechanism that may link cigarette smoking and reduced pregnancy rates following IVF is the observation that smoking appears to accelerate the rate of egg loss. Women who smoke have the elevated hormone levels that indicate a depleted supply of eggs and prematurely aged follicles.

For men, anything that may lead to atherosclerosis, such as untreated diabetes or hypertension or even health habits such as smoking and a high-fat diet, may damage blood vessels and impair blood flow, leading to impotence. A good blood supply to the penis is necessary to achieve an erection.

Marijuana has been linked to an inability to perform sexually and to diminished fertility. It also has been associated with in-

creased levels of female hormones in men and to the development
of abnormally shaped sperm. This has the effect of reducing the
production of LH and therefore decreasing the levels of the male
hormone testosterone.

Cocaine may have a negative impact on sperm development.
Recent animal experiments have shown that it damages the cells
that produce sperm.

Steroids commonly used by men to build more muscular bodies can also inhibit the ability to have a baby. Thought by some to
improve sexual performance, they actually act as a male contra-
ceptive by depressing hormone secretion and interfering with
normal sperm production.

Men should avoid using a testosterone patch, pills, or shots unless they are under a physician's supervision. In addition, men
should be aware that their use of testosterone may have the effect
of depressing or shutting off the secretion of follicle-stimulating
hormone and luteinizing hormone, which govern the production
of sperm.

In most cases, if you stop using these substances, sperm production eventually returns to normal, although it can take at least one
full cycle of sperm production—seventy-four days—before most
sperm are healthy and show up in normal amounts in your semen.

Check Out Your Medicines

A number of prescription drugs have been reported to have a negative effect on the male reproductive systems, including the ulcer
drug Tagamet (cimetidine), some antibiotics, and antihypertensive medications. For example, the use of a class of high blood
pressure medicines known as calcium channel blockers can interfere with the ability of a sperm to penetrate the outer membrane
of an egg. (See the box on page 39.)

In women, thyroid replacement therapy may affect ovulation, depending on how carefully thyroid hormones are maintained at normal levels. Ovulation may be impaired in women who have low thyroid hormone levels, so when they are on thyroid replacement therapy, the levels of pituitary hormone (which controls the thyroid) in their blood should be monitored regularly and carefully kept in the normal range.

As a couple, tell your physicians early on that you're trying to get pregnant and that you're concerned about the effects of medicines on your fertility. It's a good idea to remind your doctors about this every time they start to write a prescription for either of you.

MEDICATIONS LINKED TO MALE INFERTILITY

Chemical or Generic Name

Spironolactone is a component of several antihypertensive drugs; it may impair production of testosterone and sperm.

Sulfasalazine is found in a few medicines used for irritable bowel disease, colitis, or Crohn's disease. It adversely affects normal sperm development. Drugs with mesalamine can be substituted, instead.

Colchicine and allopurinol are used to control gout and can affect the ability of sperm to fertilize.

Antibiotics including tetracyclines, gentamicin, neomycin, erythromycin, and nitrofurantoin (in extremely high doses) can negatively affect sperm generation, movement, and density.

Cimetidine, the active ingredient in Tagamet, can sometimes cause impotence and semen abnormalities. Drugs with ranitidine and famotidine, however, do not seem to have the same effect.

Cyclosporine is used to improve graft survival in organ transplants but may have a detrimental effect on male fertility.

Be Careful with Herbal Remedies

Several popular herbal preparations probably should be added to the list of substances to avoid if you want to protect your fertility. Although many people believe that because herbs are "natural" they're safe, those that have druglike effects on the body do contain potent chemicals. Like some over-the-counter or prescription medicines, some herbal remedies may interfere with normal reproduction.

Three herbs that were tested in laboratory studies on human sperm and on hamster eggs produced adverse effects in either the sperm or the eggs, or both. Researchers at Loma Linda University School of Medicine in California have found that *tiny amounts of St. John's wort, echinacea purpurea, and ginkgo biloba made the eggs impossible or difficult to fertilize, changed the genetic material in sperm, and reduced a sperm's viability.*

The researchers pointed out that their laboratory work indicated only a potential risk. They said it was possible that people who did not exceed the recommended doses would not experience negative effects, and in the human body such doses might not actually reach eggs and sperm. However, it should be noted that, in the lab, the eggs and sperm were exposed to only minute fractions of the herbal preparations.

Blue cohosh, an herbal dietary supplement long used by some midwives and American Indians to induce labor, is also sold as a menstrual remedy and could be dangerous for women of childbearing age.

In the laboratories of the U.S. Food and Drug Administration, blue cohosh produced significant birth defects in rat embryos, such as nerve damage, twisted tails, and poor or absent eye development. The research was done in 1996–98 by Dr. Edward J. Kennelly, now at the City University of New York. The herb is also known as blueberry root, squawroot, or papooseroot.

Have Infections Treated Right Away

Women should have any vaginal or cervical infection, such as bacterial vaginosis, trichomoniasis, chlamydia, or yeast, treated immediately because the discharge may stop sperm from entering the uterus.

Men should have urinary tract infections treated promptly because some urinary tract infections, especially those involving the epididymis, may diminish long-term fertility.

Avoid Exposure to Toxins Such as Solvents and Pesticides

Studies have linked specific pesticides, chemical solvents, dusts, and other substances in the environment to instances of infertility in women and abnormal sperm or low sperm production in men.

PESTICIDES. Frequent exposure to lawn and farm chemicals can be harmful, especially those applied as a spray, because the sprays can drift some distance and be inhaled unknowingly. When using any sort of weedkillers, fungicides, or pesticides, wear a mask, long pants, long shirtsleeves, and vinyl (not latex) gloves. If you work on a farm, or in any environment where toxins may be present, you may want to invest in a mask with replaceable charcoal filters (available at hardware stores) and to wear protective clothing consistently.

DUST AND SOLVENTS. Protect yourself not only around chemicals but in situations where there's a lot of dust in the air, including dust from grains and from woodworking, particularly when the wood has been pressure-treated with preservatives. You should also wear similar protection when using volatile solvents such as paint thinners and turpentine and make certain that your work area has extremely good ventilation. To be on the safe side, this concern should apply to home projects as well.

LEAD AND X RAYS. Severe lead intoxication—seen most often among lead battery workers—can have a negative effect on both male and female reproductive systems. In addition, the reproductive organs of you and your partner should be protected against radiation when medical X rays are taken.

Men—Avoid Hot Water and Tight Pants!

The germ cells in the testicles that produce sperm work best in temperatures slightly *below* normal body temperatures. *If the temperature within the testicles is elevated by only two, three, or four degrees Fahrenheit, both sperm and testosterone production are negatively affected.* To keep the testicles cool, the scrotum (the skin sac that holds them) loosens up so that the testes are held away from the body. But if you wear tight jeans, bicycle shorts, or leather pants that hold the testicles close against your body, their temperature may rise. This also may happen if you wear undershorts made of nylon or other artificial fibers, even if they're not tight. Such fabrics hold in more heat than cotton and wool, materials that "breathe." Keeping your genital area cool also helps avoid infections that thrive in warm, moist places.

Spending time in hot tubs, Jacuzzis, and saunas, and taking long, hot showers or baths also overheat the sperm cells and may significantly impair sperm function.

___

One of the many scientists in Cambridge, Massachusetts, was fond of doing much of his thinking while having a long soak in a hot bath every day. After he and his wife had tried to conceive un-

successfully for many months, she did a little research of her own and then firmly requested that he switch to taking short, tepid showers and do his thinking elsewhere. This tactic has proved successful—they're now the parents of four children.

Maximize Your Lovemaking

Small changes in how you conduct your lovemaking can help sperm reach the uterus more easily:

- If you use a lubricant, choose it carefully. Better still, avoid them. Even though they're not designed to kill sperm, some nonspermicidal gels are gooey enough to reduce the number of sperm that get into the cervix. Even the presence of hand lotion or saliva in or near the vagina can slow down or kill sperm.
- Don't douche because it may wash out sperm you need.
- The best position for intercourse when you are trying to get pregnant is the traditional one, in which the man is positioned on top of the woman, because this allows his penis to penetrate deeply and puts the sperm close to the cervical entry to the uterus.
- After lovemaking, it's thought to be helpful if the woman lies still for twenty to thirty minutes, giving the sperm more time and opportunity to find their way into the uterus. A pillow under your hips can help the ejaculate slip toward your cervix.
- Once you know that you're ovulating, the conventional wisdom is to have intercourse every other day. There doesn't seem to be any reason, however, for not making love as often as you want during the two or three days just before and one day immediately after ovulation, when cervical mucus is re-

ceptive and your temperature chart or ovulation kit indicates that this is your fertile period. (Methods for detecting ovulation are discussed in Step 3.) However, don't feel that you need to "schedule sex"—this idea easily could have an inhibiting effect.

Learn to Reduce Stress

If possible, try to cut back at work and/or reduce the amount of traveling in your schedules for a number of months. If you can't reduce your responsibilities at work, do make a point of not taking on any extra projects at home. Tip the scales in your favor—make this a special time for the two of you to kick back and relax. Several relaxation techniques are discussed in Step 4, along with other ideas for reducing stress and being good to yourselves.

Step 2:
Maximize the Response of Your Reproductive System

The coming together of an egg and sperm is the result of two rather elaborate reproductive systems. Your fertility potential—your probability of achieving a pregnancy—is related to how well your reproductive organs are functioning and how time—and the environment—may have affected your ovaries, follicles, eggs, testes, and sperm.

THE WOMAN'S CONTRIBUTION

The process of ovulating—producing an egg—every month is a complex system that relies a great deal on the exquisite timing of the secretion of reproductive hormones. Ovulation and the fertilization of an egg result only if a series of many small but vital events occur—and at fairly precise times. As you read about this process, you may wonder how conception manages to take place at all.

How Many Eggs?

When you were born, your two ovaries already contained all the egg cells, or oocytes, you will ever have. They numbered several million in the fetal stage, were down to less than one million at the time you were born, and continued to decline in number from then on. By the time you experienced your first menstrual period, you were probably down to 250,000 eggs. However, only about 300 to 500 of these actually are released from the ovaries during the years between puberty and menopause, usually one a month from a follicle on the surface of the ovary. The number of eggs you have at the start of your reproductive life is unique to you. Medical science so far has no way of determining the number of eggs you have in your ovaries at any one time.

The problem with having all your eggs at the beginning of your life means that these delicate genetic packages will be exposed to the environmental toxins to which you're exposed. Moreover, as they age, they become less able to form a fertilized embryo that develops into a healthy infant. Unfortunately, we have no control over some of the processes that affect our eggs, although we can avoid cigarette smoking, which clearly has an aging effect on the ovaries and eggs.

As a girl approaches puberty, her body steps up the production of the hormones that make ovulation and conception possible. The most important of these hormones are estrogen, progesterone, follicle-stimulating hormone (FSH), luteinizing hormone (LH), and gonadotropin-releasing hormone (GnRH).

Normal ovulation depends on a sequence of events that starts off as nerve signals in your brain. These are converted into hormonal signals by a walnut-size area in your brain called the hypothalamus, which produces pulses of gonadotropin-releasing hormone every sixty to ninety minutes. GnRH stimulates the nearby pituitary gland to secrete FSH and then LH at certain times in your ovulatory cycle. These two hormones are called gonadotropins because in both sexes they affect the gonads—the ovaries and the testicles.

In response to FSH, several follicles (tiny, fluid-filled sacs in the ovary that each contain an oocyte) enlarge and their egg cells mature. Only one of these follicles becomes dominant and is able to ovulate, which is why most human pregnancies result in one child. Then, at midcycle, a surge of LH prompts the release of the egg from the largest follicle. This egg is gathered up by the nearest fallopian tube where, if healthy sperm have arrived, fertilization may take place.

The Female Reproductive System (side view)

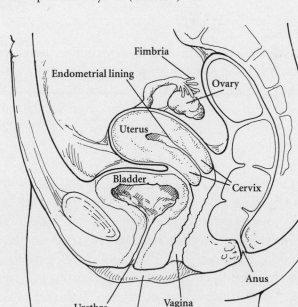

The Female Reproductive System (front view)

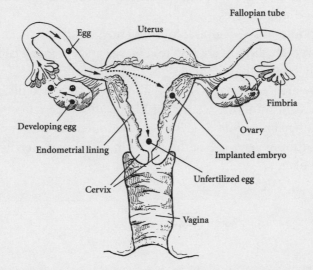

For this cycle of events to occur every month, however, you need a normally functioning hormone system, healthy ovaries capable of growing an egg, and an open fallopian tube.

The Menstrual Cycle—Day by Day

Day 1 of your menstrual cycle is the first day of menstruation, which takes place because no fertilized egg implanted in your uterus in the previous cycle. The two hormones—estradiol (estrogen) and progesterone—were secreted to prepare your uterus for an implantation. Because they were not needed their levels dropped sharply, causing the thickened, blood-rich endometrium layer of the uterus to be sloughed off as menstrual blood.

As you begin to menstruate, the pituitary once again releases FSH to stimulate an ovarian follicle to enlarge. We don't yet understand why in an individual woman certain follicles—almost always one—will react to the increasing pulses of FSH stimulation.

We do know that in most women some follicles will enlarge in response to FSH. Furthermore, one follicle almost always will produce more estrogen than the others, and becomes the dominant follicle that releases an egg around day 14 of the cycle. The presence of FSH also will cause these follicles to make estradiol, which enters your bloodstream, circulates to your brain, and resets your hypothalamus and pituitary gland, modulating the amounts of FSH and LH they secrete in the following days.

The Menstrual Cycle

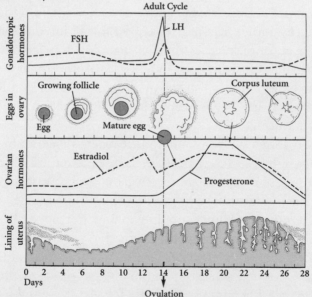

This chart illustrates the events of the menstrual cycle. During the first half, luteinizing hormone (LH) and follicle-stimulating hormone (FSH) are secreted at steady levels and stimulate the ovary to produce a mature egg. At midcycle, surges of both LH and FSH cause an ovarian follicle to release the egg (ovulation). FSH and LH then drop to their baseline levels. After ovulation, the follicle turns into a cystlike body called the corpus luteum, which produces progesterone. Increasing levels of estradiol, a type of estrogen made by the follicles during the midcycle, and progesterone together promote endometrial growth in the uterus for possible egg implantation. If the egg is not fertilized or doesn't implant, the levels of progesterone and estradiol decline, the endometrium is sloughed off, and menstruation begins.

The process of follicle enlargement, egg maturation, and the release of the egg is the result of a frequently shifting balance among your hormones. Your reproductive hormones must be present in your bloodstream at the right levels and at the right times for ovulation to take place.

DAYS 8–10. Between days 8 and 10 the dominant follicle becomes so large it easily can be seen by ultrasound. Although the egg itself is too small to be visualized, it is maturing within the follicle and becoming capable of being fertilized. In the cell stage, an egg contains all the pairs of chromosomes that normal cells possess. It remains at this state of genetic development until the cell is stimulated by a midcycle surge of LH. At this point, one set of the paired chromosomes leaves the cell, forming a polar body just outside the cell wall. This body of leftover chromosomal material, which can be seen under a strong microscope, is used by infertility laboratories during IVF procedures as a sign that an egg is successfully maturing.

DAYS 12–13. As the dominant follicle reaches maximum size by day 12 or 13, it is secreting peak levels of estrogen which, among other actions, sensitizes the pituitary gland to the pulses of GnRH from the hypothalamus. In response, the pituitary releases that important burst of stored-up luteinizing hormone. It is this timely LH surge, plus the many interactions of other hormones within the follicle, that regulates its growth, the growth of the egg, and finally, the egg's release. Within twenty-four to thirty-six hours after the LH surge reaches the follicle, it ruptures and its fluids ooze out, carrying along the egg. This is ovulation.

The empty follicle now turns into a yellowish, cystlike body called the corpus luteum. During the second half of your ovulatory cycle, the corpus luteum continues to make estrogen and also secretes progesterone.

Fertilization

Surrounded by a cloud of sticky cumulus cells that developed during the hours before ovulation, the egg lies on the surface of the ovary. One end of each fallopian tube is connected to your uterus and the other end, which looks somewhat like a funnel, is near the ovary and is open. This opening is edged with hundreds of little fingerlike projections called fimbria. A healthy fallopian tube has fine muscles that enable it to bend toward the ovary, where the egg's sticky exterior makes it relatively easy for the fimbria to gather it into the fallopian tube. The egg will stay at the funnel end of the fallopian tube for one or two days, and it's here that sperm most often reaches it and fertilization takes place. No one knows exactly how long an egg can live outside its follicle, but laboratory research suggests that fertilization usually occurs within twenty-four to thirty-six hours after ovulation.

Although a normal ovulation process is an important part of attaining a pregnancy, it's not the whole story. A sperm still has to be able to reach the egg and fertilize it, and the resulting embryo has to be moved into the uterus and become implanted.

The Cervix Gets Ready

The high levels of estradiol produced by the dominant follicle just before ovulation prepare your cervix for the passage of sperm. Sperm can't traverse the cervix unless the right kind of mucus is present. As your estradiol levels increase, the cervix produces a kind of mucus that looks and feels somewhat like slippery egg white and its opening (os) relaxes and widens. This combination of events makes it easier for many sperm to move swiftly out of the vagina into your uterus and up into the fallopian tubes.

This so-called fertile mucus serves many functions. It protects sperm from the normally acidic vaginal secretions which usually kill them within a few hours. And for some sperm the protective mucus of the cervix provides a place to wait for one or two days before they continue their journey into the uterus and toward the fallopian tubes. Why some sperm move quickly into the uterus and others linger behind is still an unsolved mystery.

If the mucus-producing glands in your cervix don't work properly or if your estrogen levels are not sufficiently high, not enough fertile mucus will be produced. Moreover, there is only a narrow window of time—up to seven days—in each cycle in which such mucus is made.

The main task of the progesterone from the corpus luteum is to prepare the lining of the uterus to accept the embryo. Additionally, within a few days after ovulation, the progesterone causes the cervix to tighten and its mucus to become so thick and sticky that it blocks sperm from entering. It's estimated that flaws in cervical functioning may be factors in 5 to 10 percent of all infertility cases.

If you have intercourse while the cervical mucus is in its welcoming form, normal, active sperm can quickly reach the fallopian tubes. If an egg is present, one sperm works its way through the egg's protective covering, the zona pellucida, which then changes chemically and permits no other sperm to enter. (More details on this process are in the following section.) This prevents the genetic mix-up that would occur if the chromosomes of more than one sperm combined with the chromosomes of the egg.

Mature sperm have twenty-three chromosomes, and although eggs start out with forty-six, after LH stimulation half of the original complement of chromosomes leave the egg cell. Eggs contain an X chromosome and sperm contain either an X or Y chromosome, the so-called sex chromosomes. When a sperm fertilizes an egg, its twenty-three chromosomes (with either an X or Y) combine with the egg's twenty-three chromosomes, so a fertilized egg has a full, normal complement of forty-six chromosomes. Through this process the embryo will possess equal portions of its parents' genetic material. If that particular sperm is carrying the Y chromosome, the egg will develop into a male embryo because the Y provides all the information for the development of male sexual characteristics. If the sperm carries an X chromosome, the embryo will follow a female pattern.

After the genetic materials from sperm and egg join, the egg develops into an embryo and begins to divide. In older eggs, however, it is during this early stage that the mechanism of gene replication may not function correctly, genetic disorders may occur, and the embryo may fail to develop.

Implantation

The fallopian tube moves what now has become a microscopic embryo toward the uterus, using its hairlike cilia to "wave" it along. If cilia are not present, or too few exist, the embryo may not move and may implant into the wall of the tube, causing a tubal (ectopic) pregnancy. If your tubes have been damaged by infection, surgery, or other trauma, the embryo may not be able to get through and become either a tubal pregnancy or die from lack of nutritional support.

Implantation in the Uterus

While all this has been going on, the lining of your uterus—the endometrium—has been getting ready to nurture an embryo. The high estradiol and progesterone levels secreted by the corpus luteum induce the endometrium to become thick and spongy, and to grow new blood vessels for nourishing an implanted embryo. For the embryo to attach itself it must break out of its zona pellucida membrane, an event appropriately dubbed hatching.

Once hatched, most embryos settle into a nook in the endometrium and, within a few days, hook up with its microscopic blood vessels. After this connection is made, what is now the outermost membrane around the cell cluster, the chorion, begins to secrete human chorionic gonadotropin (hCG). About the tenth day after ovulation, hCG can be detected in your blood. However, its presence doesn't indicate whether the embryo is in the uterus or in a fallopian tube.

Your Immune Response and Your Embryo

Some women conceive without difficulty, yet repeatedly lose their pregnancies. A small number (some 5 percent) of these miscarriages may be due to an immunity factor.

In general, if cells with a genetic composition different from ours are injected into our bodies, our immune systems reject and attack them because they are foreign. In a pregnancy, the embryo is detected at first by the mother's immune system as different cell tissue and the rejection process is started. The embryo then signals the mother's immune system that it's meant to be in the uterus. Her immune system responds by producing antibodies and other proteins designed to protect the embryo throughout the pregnancy.

For your body to produce such protective antibodies, it must first perceive your embryo to be something foreign. This may not always take place. One theory used to explain frequent miscarriages is that if a couple is too closely related or if the tissues of their bodies are very much alike, they may produce embryos that are too similar to the mother's genetic makeup to be recognized as foreign, and the necessary antibodies aren't elicited.

Starting Over

The corpus luteum continues to secrete estrogen and progesterone for fourteen days after a woman has ovulated. If an embryo
hasn't implanted by day 23 or 24, the levels of these hormones
drop rapidly, the endometrium breaks up, menstruation starts,
and the ovulatory cycle starts again.

THE MAN'S CONTRIBUTION

A man's hypothalamus, like the woman's, releases regular pulses
of GnRH. In his case, these prompt his pituitary to secrete pulses
of follicle-stimulating hormone and luteinizing hormone. In a
man, FSH stimulates the Sertoli cells in the testicles and drives the
germ cells to make sperm; the LH triggers the testicles' Leydig cells
to produce the male hormone testosterone, which gives a man his
masculine appearance and sex drive and helps sperm mature.
Sperm are formed in the testicles and mature in the epididymis
before being expelled through the penis during ejaculation. A
boy's body becomes capable of performing this process toward
the end of puberty, usually between the ages of twelve to sixteen.

The Male Reproductive System (side view)

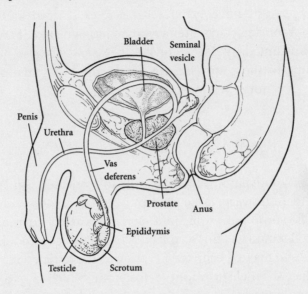

Testicles are formed in the male abdomen and, by birth, have descended into the scrotum, the pouch of skin that holds them outside the body. If testicles fail to descend or don't develop completely, this often—but not always—may reduce sperm production and be a source of infertility. At maturity, each testicle is about 1.5 inches long by 1 inch wide. In many men, it's normal for one testicle to be larger than the other, and one testicle may be higher in the scrotum than the other.

The scrotum's function is to keep the testicles at the right temperature for making sperm. Because the testicles are suspended outside the body, their usual temperature is two degrees cooler than the body's internal temperature. When outside temperatures are cold, the scrotum tightens up to hold the testicles snug against the body to keep them warm. When the testicle temperature is too high, the scrotum becomes very loose, exposing them to more air.

However, the scrotum can't counteract extreme temperature effects, such as those caused by a long soak in a hot bath or Jacuzzi. Testes exposed to high temperatures produce fewer sperm and sperm that don't appear normal or move very vigorously. It takes about two and a half months for the effects of an exposure to extreme heat to wear off.

Making Sperm

FSH stimulates the Sertoli cells to provide nutrients so that sperm cells (spermatocytes) will grow. After puberty, young men constantly produce sperm cells, about a thousand per second. Over a seventy-four-day period these spermatocytes will develop into sperm with heads that contain their genetic material, middle sections that provide their energy for rapid movement, and long, whiplike tails for propelling themselves.

To finish their growth process, maturing sperm float into the epididymis, a tightly coiled set of ultra-fine tubes that you can feel along the back of each testicle. Here they finish their maturation process, become able to move under their own power, and move into the vas deferens, the duct that carries sperm from the epididymis to the urethra, where they remain until ejaculation.

Close-up of a Sperm

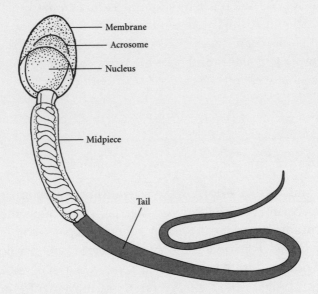

Sperm Quality

Of the millions of sperm the average man produces every day, about 40 percent will be imperfect. They may have abnormally shaped heads or more than one head or be missing part of their genetic material. Because sperm formation is not a perfect process, this is one reason you make so many sperm. Furthermore, normal sperm can be damaged by infections in your reproductive system.

A man's ejaculate, a mixture of sperm and semen, contains two to six milliliters of fluid (about ⅓ to 1 teaspoon); each milliliter contains 20 to 200 million sperm. (Semen is fluid from the seminal vesicles and prostate; it stimulates sperm motility.) Some men whose ejaculate commonly contains fewer than 20 million sperm per cubic centimeter of ejaculate experience impaired fertility to some degree. Many men whose ejaculate has fewer than 5 million total motile sperm have significantly diminished fertility.

The Last Leg of the Journey

The vas deferens duct carries sperm from the epididymis to the urethra. During orgasm sperm pass through the prostate, and seminal fluid from that gland mixes with them in the prostate section of the urethra, forming the ejaculate that holds the sperm together. The male urethra has two functions. When you urinate, it transports urine from the bladder. During intercourse it carries ejaculate. When you're aroused, the opening between the bladder and urethra closes to prevent urine from joining the semen. Afterward, it takes a short time for this system to reverse itself so that you can urinate.

During orgasm your pelvic muscles, prostate, and the muscular lining of the vas deferens tighten, forcing semen down the urethra and out the penis. Each ejaculate normally contains tens of millions of sperm.

As we mentioned, if intercourse takes place close to the time of ovulation, the mucus produced by the woman's cervix is of a consistency that allows sperm to swim through it. Many sperm that pass through the mucus move quickly into the uterus and up through the fallopian tubes within five to ten minutes. Speed is important because sperm survival in the cervix and reproductive tract is only about forty-eight hours.

If the fallopian tubes are unobstructed, the sperm swim swiftly toward the egg, assisted by tubal contractions and enticed by chemical and hormonal signals emanating from the egg. When hundreds of sperm begin swarming all over the egg in their urge to enter it, they inevitably interact with its masses of cumulus cells and, apparently, release an enzyme that breaks down those cells.

Within a few hours, thousands of sperm have died during this on-slaught, but the cumulus has fallen away and the zona pellucida of the egg is exposed. Hundreds of sperm attach themselves to this protective covering, one finally penetrates it, and the zona pellu-cida closes up to further penetration.

The Acrosome Reaction

Researchers have long wondered what was different or better about the single sperm that was able to outdo hundreds of others and get through the zona pellucida. What's now known is that a sperm has to be "activated" to be able to accomplish this. The head of the sperm not only contains the chromosomes but is also sheathed in what is called the acrosome membrane. Before a sperm can penetrate an egg, certain enzymes in the acrosome membrane must be turned on—the necessary acrosome reaction. The activated enzymes bore into the zona pellucida, allowing the sperm to enter the egg. Abnormalities in any aspect of the acro-some reaction may be a source of male infertility.

As the sperm fuses with the egg, its chromosomes join the egg's and form a cell that's a new genetic package. This cell then divides again and again, every sixteen hours or so, and the new arrange-ment of chromosomes is duplicated in each new cell. This multi-plying cluster of cells moves down the fallopian tube and enters the uterus. If it implants itself successfully in the endometrium, it will spend the next thirty-seven weeks being nourished, first by the enriched endometrium and then by the placenta, an organ also rich in blood vessels that provides what is now a growing fe-tus with the oxygen and nutrients necessary to nourish it until it's born.

Step 3:
Target Possible Problems

Since problems with ovulation or sperm production are the most common causes of infertility, it makes sense to look at these functions first.

Every month a woman's body offers several clues that say she's ovulating: regular, often uncomfortable menstrual periods, premenstrual breast fullness and tenderness, changes in the amount and quality of cervical mucus, and perhaps the brief abdominal cramping or pain between periods that may indicate the release of an egg. Women who menstruate regularly—having periods every twenty-eight to thirty-two days—don't often have an ovulation problem.

ARE YOU OVULATING?

There are three techniques you can use to discover when—and if—in your cycle you actually ovulate: the *cervical mucus method*, the *basal body temperature (BBT) method*, and *urine LH testing*, which means using an ovulation kit to test your urine for luteinizing hormone, the hormone that triggers the release of an egg from the ovary.

The Cervical Mucus Method

This technique takes advantage of the fact that the secretions from your cervix change during your ovulatory cycle. A few days before the egg leaves the ovary, the high estrogen levels in your blood cause your cervical mucus to become more abundant. You're likely to be more aware of its presence even before you check it with your fingers. It looks clear and feels slippery and stretchy. You may even be able to stretch it for a couple of inches between thumb and forefinger. The presence of this mucus (often called fertile-type mucus) is a sign that ovulation is about to take place. Checking the texture and quantity of your cervical mucus every day and noting on your calendar or your temperature chart the presence or absence of fertile mucus costs nothing and is easy to do. Combining a cervical mucus check with a record of your daily basal body temperature for a couple of months can easily give you a pretty good picture of your ovulatory cycle, including when in the cycle you are ovulating.

Charting Your Basal Body Temperature

Your basal body temperature (BBT) is your resting temperature in the morning before you get out of bed. A day or two before ovulation it may drop a few tenths of a degree. After the egg has left the ovary, your temperature rises about half a degree and remains at that level for the next twelve to fourteen days. It again drops slightly just before menstruation; if it doesn't, you may be running a fever—or you may be pregnant.

Sample Chart

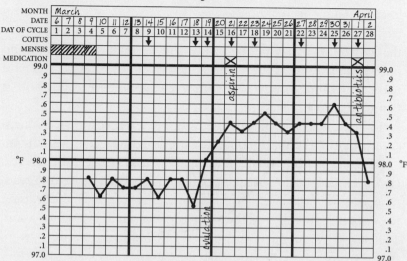

Instructions for Keeping a Basal Body Temperature Chart

1. Use only a special "metabolic" thermometer with a Fahrenheit scale, available at your local pharmacy. Learn to read it accurately.

2. Shake down the thermometer before you go to bed and place it on your bedside table.

3. Take your temperature each morning immediately after waking, before rising, eating, drinking, smoking, or undertaking any type of physical activity. Temperature should be taken for five minutes, by the clock. Record your temperature as a solid dot at the intersection of the appropriate temperature and date lines on the BBT chart. Cycle day 1 is the first day of menstruation.

4. Indicate, in the appropriate places, when intercourse and menstruation occur. Also note on the chart any potential reasons for temperature variation such as illness, infection, and insomnia. Also be sure to place an *x* on the medication line and write in the name of any medication, such as aspirin, acetaminophen, antihistamine, or antibiotic, taken during the month.

5. Your BBT is an indirect predictor that cannot pinpoint the exact day of ovulation. Therefore, it is important to have sexual intercourse at the anticipated time of ovulation. Ideally, intercourse should take place at least every other day beginning two to four days prior to the anticipated day of ovulation. This is your most fertile period.

6. Start a new chart when menstrual bleeding begins.

Changes in your BBT reveal quite a bit about your cycle. If your BBT follows the two-stage pattern of a lower temperature followed by a higher reading for ten to fourteen days, you can feel fairly confident that you are ovulating. If it doesn't stay high for that period, you may not be producing enough progesterone and have what is called a luteal phase defect. If your temperature remains the same throughout your cycle, ovulation might not be taking place.

To be able to rely on this method, however, you need to measure your BBT carefully. Since your temperature changes as soon as you start moving in the morning, you need to take it before you get out of bed. Because regular thermometers can be hard to read, especially when you're half asleep, buy a special BBT thermometer, which registers only the temperature range between 95 and 100 degrees Fahrenheit and clearly shows fractional changes in temperature. These thermometers are available at drugstores and cost approximately $12 to $15. For accuracy, shake it down to 96 degrees the night before and put it next to your bed.

It's vital to take your BBT before you get out of bed, talk, or drink anything, even a glass of water. You must also have had at least three hours' sleep to get an accurate reading. You can record your BBT if you wake up in the night, as long as you've already had three hours' sleep and you take your temperature before you get out of bed. You can use the thermometer orally, rectally, or vaginally as long as you use the same method every time. Leave the thermometer in place for as long as its instructions dictate, usually about five minutes.

Monthly charts for noting each day's BBT are available from your doctor and from family planning clinics, or you can use ordinary graph paper. A change in your BBT of only a fraction of a degree is important. Mark each tenth of a degree with a dot on your chart; connecting the dots will make it easier to see the day-to-day changes. Your chart may contain some unexpected blips that represent a sleepless night or an emotional upset, but these generally don't affect the overall pattern. If you have an unusually high or low reading any morning and you can figure out the reason, write that on the chart.

Several events other than ovulation can cause a rise in your BBT. Illness accompanied by a fever can cause variations in your current cycle *and in the next one.* A low-grade infection, a cold, or the flu can lead to a rise of a few tenths of a degree, enough to affect your BBT. Drinking alcohol, including wine or beer, in the evening may cause a rise in your BBT the next morning. Taking your temperature later than usual in the morning, even if you haven't gotten out of bed, may also produce a higher reading. When these things happen, note it on the chart in case there's a temperature deviation.

After several months of recording your daily BBT, you should see a pattern of one, two, or three low-temperature days approximately in the middle of your cycle. These are the prelude to ovulation, and usually are followed by a slight but definite rise in temperature that occurs after the egg leaves the ovary. Because the temperature rise is triggered by progesterone from the corpus luteum, *after* the egg leaves the follicle, the BBT method can't be used as an *advance* warning of ovulation. What it does, however, is demonstrate whether you are ovulating and where in your cycle ovulation takes place. Because your BBT can be affected easily by emotional disturbances or illness, it's wise to track it for two or three months for greatest accuracy.

Ovulation Test Kits

Unlike a BBT chart, a urine test can alert you to ovulation that's getting ready to happen, so you can time your lovemaking accordingly. You use these commercial kits a few days before the midpoint of your cycle to check for the presence of luteinizing hormone (LH) in your urine. As we mentioned in Step 2, a surge of this hormone prompts the release of the mature egg from the ovary within approximately thirty-six hours. The presence of LH in your urine is a clear signal that ovulation is about to take place. If you've been charting your BBT or checking your cervical mucus every day, you'll have a good idea of when in your cycle ovulation is likely to occur, and when you can start testing your urine.

Ovulation test kits are available in most drugstores and discount stores. They cost as little as $15 for a store brand for morning urine to about $70 for the only one that will test afternoon urine. For the most accurate results, you should repeat the test in successive months, especially if you find no evidence of ovulation. Sickness or long air trips across several time zones can affect your ovulatory cycle.

The instructions will tell you on what day of your cycle to begin testing, how to collect and test your urine, and what the results mean. Most kits are designed for checking your first morning urine for five or six days for the presence of LH. They're not all alike, and convenience of design varies from brand to brand, so read the directions and compare kits before you buy to find the one that will be the easiest for you to use.

WHAT'S THE STATE OF YOUR SPERM?

In addition to discovering what the woman's ovulatory cycle is like, the appearance, vigor, and density of the man's sperm should be determined. It isn't necessary to postpone sperm evaluation until after you've been trying to conceive for twelve months or until the possibility of an ovulation problem has been explored, although some fertility specialists may suggest this. Performing sperm tests right away can save time and help to reduce apprehension and anxiety. Adequate sperm testing can take almost as long as developing an ovulation profile. Urologists who specialize in infertility suggest that at least three semen analyses be made to establish a baseline picture of sperm health. If there's any question about the findings, more sophisticated testing may be necessary.

For the male, the evaluation for fertility should include a complete medical history and a physical examination, in addition to the pertinent laboratory tests. It is not unusual for the medical history or physical examination to reveal the source of an infertility problem.

How to Get a Good Sperm Specimen

To obtain a good-quality semen specimen, you should collect it after you haven't ejaculated for two or three days, and it should be brought directly to the laboratory that will be doing the analysis within two hours after ejaculation. For the sake of accuracy, it's important to collect each sample after the same interval of abstinence. The best container is a wide-mouthed glass jar that is clean but not necessarily sterile.

Semen can be collected by masturbation, coitus interruptus, or by using a condom that isn't made with a spermicide. Masturbation is the method preferred for most accurate results. Put your name, date, the time the semen was collected, and the length of the abstinence period on the jar. On your way to the lab, don't let the specimen get cold. Keep it next to your body under your clothes if at all possible.

Just as you want to choose a urologist who has a great deal of experience with infertility patients, you also want to make certain the lab testing your semen sample performs this work frequently, not just a couple of times a month. Ask your urologist or the laboratory about how common it is for the lab to run semen tests. To get an accurate answer from the lab, ask to speak to the director or the chief laboratory technician.

Checking the Health of Your Sperm

For a sperm to do its job, it needs to be able to penetrate cervical mucus, move rapidly through the female reproductive tract, bore into the membrane around the egg, and fertilize it. In analyzing a semen sample, the instrument that counts the sperm also determines how many of them are active, and how fast they are able to move. To accomplish this, most laboratories today use computer-assisted semen analysis, or CASA.

The shape of your sperm also is important because it reveals whether your sperm-producing capability is working all right and whether your sperm can perform the considerable task of getting to the egg and fertilizing it. Sperm with abnormal-looking heads are less likely to be able to move or, if they can, move more slowly than they should. Sperm need to have normally shaped heads to be able to pass through the channels in the cervical mucus, bind to the egg, and penetrate it.

If the analysis of your semen reveals a low number of sperm, lack of vigorous movement, or abnormal shapes, further testing may be needed to pinpoint more precisely where the problem may lie. The selection of further tests, if any, should be left to the judgment of a urologist experienced in infertility.

Step 4:
Ease Emotional Stress:
The Harvard Behavioral Medicine Program for Infertility

Is there an infertility patient anywhere who hasn't wondered about the connection between stress and infertility? Or who hasn't heard that well-meaning but infuriating comment: "You're just too tense. Relax and you'll get pregnant." Or been told: "Just adopt and you're bound to get pregnant . . . or perhaps you should quit your job." However thoughtless they may be, these comments do not come out of nowhere—stress and infertility have been linked since biblical times. In the Book of Samuel it was written that a woman named Hannah was so grieved over her childlessness she couldn't stop weeping. After many years of sadness, she told a priest of her torment; he said words of comfort to her and a year later she gave birth to a son who grew up to become Samuel the Prophet.

The main focus of infertility researchers during the past three or four decades has been on medical or surgical solutions to infertility; however, during this same period some researchers did observe a connection between stress and infertility. For a long time, however, it wasn't clear which came first—the infertility or the psychological distress associated with it—and what the mechanism of the relationship was. There also were some unresolved questions about the definition of "stress" itself. Today, fortunately, we know a lot more: we recognize that infertility is one of the most stressful events in a person's life, that the relationship between emotions and infertility is very real and very complex, and that stress—and the accompanying feelings of anxiety and depression—contribute to some cases of infertility. We also have a better idea of how our emotions physically affect our reproductive systems.

A number of studies have found significantly more anxiety and depression in infertile women than in those who are fertile. Their depression scores are very much like those of women who have cancer, heart disease, or HIV. Almost 11 percent of infertile women meet the psychological criteria for a current, major depressive episode. Infertile women usually state that infertility is the worst crisis of their lives, that it's even worse than divorce or the death of a parent.

Such comparisons may seem extreme until you consider all the ramifications of the infertility experience. What other medical condition has such a negative effect on a couple's relationship since men and women react so differently to infertility? Or on their sex life? Or on their relationship with their families and friends, especially when their siblings and friends begin to have children and their lives then revolve around those children?

Furthermore, infertility often affects a couple's jobs since certain treatments require a daily morning visit to the doctor's office, and treatment cycles may mean that business travel must be postponed or given up. For both, taking time off for frequent doctors' appointments may even raise the question of job security. Money is likely to be another worry because few insurance policies adequately cover infertility treatments, if they pay for them at all. Even a couple's religious beliefs may become a problem. Instead of being a comfort, some religions prohibit certain infertility treatments and partners may not agree on the importance of obeying those rules.

What compounds such distress is the fact that the urge to reproduce is one of the strongest in the animal kingdom. The reproducing instinct is stronger than the instinct to survive. As you may know, in many species, the male will die for the chance to mate and females will die to protect their young. It should come as no surprise that infertile individuals, particularly women, experience acute distress when they fear they may not have the family they've always wanted and expected to have.

EMOTIONS YOU MAY FACE

Although the stress levels for most couples who are struggling with infertility peak somewhere between the second and third year of trying to get pregnant, some of the anxieties associated with this difficult period of life can show up earlier than you expect and catch you completely off guard.

The first might be a lack of certainty about your desire to have a baby. Bringing a child into your life is an irreversible act. Despite all the jokes, you can't send the baby back if you find you don't like being a parent. Even while you're using ovulation kits, you may be worrying about whether you'll be able to handle the twenty-four-hour responsibility of a baby. Trying to make this decision can be one of the first major stresses. In fact, just *thinking* about having a child can be anxiety-provoking.

Men and Women Behave Differently

Another common cause of depression in women and a major cause of stress in a marriage is the fact that men and women do not always react the same way to events and often deal with their emotions very differently. For example, you may tend to become obsessed with your menstrual cycle and the fact it recurs when you're hoping it won't. Menstruation, perhaps once greeted with a sigh of relief, now is likely to become a source of tears and concern: What's wrong with me? Why is my body doing this to me? And while you're feeling traumatized, and want to talk about your fears, you're likely to discover that your husband isn't feeling the same way. He may be sympathetic because you're upset, but he doesn't really understand your feelings. And his response to your tears may be infuriating: "That's too bad, honey, but don't worry about it—it'll probably happen next month. Should we get takeout for dinner?"

We know men and women are different, but why this big discrepancy in important feelings? What mental health professionals have learned is that men just are not programmed to feel as women do about childbearing. Because a man cannot get pregnant, he is not—and is never likely to be—as emotionally invested in the ability to get pregnant. *We cannot emphasize enough that this difference in feelings between men and women is normal and quite common.*

GRACE'S STORY

I got married when I was thirty-eight, and although I knew intellectually that it might be difficult for me to get pregnant, I didn't really believe it. I've been told that my ovaries have aged so much that we have to face the real possibility of failing at this. My husband is younger than I am and my fear is that I've failed him and I've failed our marriage because I've kept him from being a father. In fact, I asked him if he wants to leave. He said he didn't. He loves me.

What's been good for us is that, thanks to the classes, we're learning to work through this situation. We've had to look at every path we could take, so for us this has turned out to be a journey. Right now we're looking at using donated eggs. I thought doing this would really be going over the top, but my husband wants to consider it. So I've learned to work through my concerns and he's learning why I cry all the time and to accept my need to tell people how I feel. We didn't talk like this before and now we're sharing our feelings, instead of him always being on the outside.

I'm still crying a lot—anything that reminds me of a baby makes me cry. I feel I'm grieving for the biological child I can't have. For a long time I told myself—and everyone—that I don't have a problem, next month I'm sure I'll get pregnant. If I just ignore it it'll happen. Now, for the first time, I'm allowing myself to recognize my feelings, to be depressed. I'm learning to come to terms with being unable to have a baby from one of my eggs.

If the reason for your infertility is a male factor—that the male partner has a problem in his reproductive system—the emotional pain he feels can be as intense as any infertile woman's. Whether he's able to talk about it, however, depends very much on the individual man.

Whether your infertility is the result of a male or female factor or problems with both your reproductive systems, it may be helpful to remember that, from boyhood, many men have been conditioned not to cry. Your male partner may be afraid to give way to his feelings, for fear of being unmanly or of losing control of himself or the situation. He may never have liked verbalizing about emotions or emotional subjects and, unlike you, he might not find comfort in ventilating his feelings. He may feel that every relationship needs a strong person and that's his role (although he may not tell you that!). In addition, he'd rather "do something" about a problem. If he feels you both are already doing everything you can, then he'd rather talk about something else.

Furthermore, he may fear that talking about infertility or its possibility will make you even sadder—and more emotional. For these reasons, and because he doesn't understand how talking through emotions could be helpful for you, he may avoid the subject or withdraw when you bring it up. If you interpret this as a lack of concern, it's likely to make you angry and the situation worse.

What can exacerbate this state of affairs is that this may be your first serious crisis as a couple. You may not yet have developed coping skills or the ability to discuss or negotiate severe conflicts in your relationship. You may not have discussed how you each respond differently to various predicaments or learned how to have relatively calm talks about highly charged issues.

The stress between you can be severely compounded if one of you already has a child. The assumption then may be made, almost automatically, that any infertility is the other person's fault, with both of you forgetting that fertility could be a sometime thing.

Emotional Pressures on the Man

Although he may not be as psychologically invested in achieving a pregnancy as a woman may be, the man who cannot impregnate his partner must deal with many of the same emotions as an infertile woman. He may feel guilty about denying her the opportunity to have a child. He may wonder whether his past sexual behavior or carelessness about his health might be the cause of his infertility. And he must cope with his emotional responses to treatment while at the same time he is trying to live up to the world's (and his own) view that he is the calm, strong person in the relationship.

In addition, even the most modern man is likely to feel less like a man if he cannot impregnate his partner. It can be difficult for some men to separate manliness (being potent) from infertility. His brothers and friends are all fathering babies—why can't he? He may prefer to assume that it's not his fault, an attitude some urologists call the Henry VIII syndrome. If he's faced with the fact that his sperm count is low, he may feel shame, and he may not be able to talk about such feelings.

Just because he doesn't want to discuss it—or doesn't know how to comfort his partner—doesn't mean that a man's emotional response is any less painful. It just may be different.

When Your Support System Lets You Down

Another source of sadness when you can't get pregnant is what *doesn't happen* when you want to discuss it with your friends and your family. Your mother, who probably was never infertile, is sure you'll eventually get pregnant and can't understand why you're so worried. Your father doesn't even want to talk about it. And, in all probability, your siblings and your friends are so busy being pregnant and trying to manage the particular stresses of coping with small children they can't begin to empathize with you. In fact, they may wonder aloud how you possibly can complain since your life is so carefree compared to theirs. You feel you've become the odd one out. It's a lonely feeling, and it's happening just when you really need to talk to someone.

As months pass and you're still not pregnant, you may be surprised how angry and jealous you feel when you see someone who is pregnant or has a baby, or if you just hear about someone else's pregnancy. And because you are of childbearing age, you are likely to be surrounded by evidence of others' fertility.

For many women trying to get pregnant, being with pregnant women or with infants becomes intolerable. You may find yourself avoiding family gatherings and social events with your friends because they're likely to include children. If you have a night out with friends who have begun their families, it seems as if they can't talk about anything except children, even when they know you're struggling with infertility.

After going home depressed from too many such occasions, it's not unusual for infertile couples, particularly infertile women, to withdraw from their usual social lives, even to the point where they cease to chat on the telephone with anyone who has a child. As a result, they feel more isolated and "different" than ever from persons who once were part of their support system.

ALEXANDRA'S STORY

I'm only thirty years old and I've been infertile for two years. I still can't believe it. My mother and sister had no trouble getting pregnant, and I'd been so careful for so long not to get pregnant that sometimes my infertility just doesn't seem possible. I find myself being mad at the world—why should other people be able to have babies and not me? There are all those people who say they don't want children and yet they have them, and I can't. What makes it worse is that there's no explanation for my problem. I'm so angry and I have no real focus for my anger.

Every time I have a failed cycle and every time one of my friends gets pregnant I have these feelings of resentment and frustration. I'm used to being successful in difficult areas and I always believed that if you work hard you succeed. That makes it hard for me to accept that I can't accomplish this. I've built my whole future on being a mother. I get so depressed that I even wonder if I'll keep my married friends or whether they'll ostracize me.

I spend my whole day feeling keyed up. And it seems as if I spend half my life counting off cycle days. Being an infertility patient is like having a part-time job—there are medical appoint-

ments, lab work; I can't travel or even attend some meetings be-cause I have to see the doctor on specific days. In fact, both my hus-band and I have this problem. There are things we can't schedule at our jobs because we have to be available for intrauterine insem-ination. And then there's the difficulty of explaining this to our bosses. What really gets to me, however, is that my boss talks about her toddlers almost nonstop.

If having a family is something we can't achieve, it's really go-ing to be hard for me. I always dreamt I'd be a mother. But, you know, what's even harder is not knowing when it will end. Not to have a definite time when you can step back into normal life again and be the person you were before.

Besides tangible events that are severely distressing, the infertile woman's own thoughts can exacerbate her feelings of failure and grief. Women are quick to blame themselves for their infertility, feeling guilty about earlier sexual relationships, or an abortion, or having used an IUD for contraception.

When Your Church or Your God Lets You Down

During this difficult period your faith in God may be shaken se-verely. If you've believed in the efficacy of prayer and feel that your prayers usually are answered, to have unexplained infertility con-tinue or treatments fail can leave you feeling angry at God and even more depressed, anxious, and alone.

Furthermore, some religious denominations may discourage or forbid an assisted reproduction procedure. The most common prohibition appears to be the use of IVF (in vitro fertilization), which is forbidden by the Catholic Church because in this proce-dure conception occurs outside the sexual act. The church views

IVF as a replacement for the conjugal act between husband and wife—a replacement that is contrary to the dignity of the couple, the marriage, and the child who may result. For many women, it's a shock and a source of grief to discover that their religion forbids the only procedure that may resolve their infertility.

When you are already distressed, not having your prayers answered or being in conflict with your religious institution can add immensely to your emotional burden. Your spiritual connection with God—the mainstay you probably never questioned—is failing you now just when you most need its support. If you and your husband decide to go ahead with the forbidden procedure, you may feel you have to leave your church. Or your anger at not having your prayers answered also can make you want to abandon your faith in a loving, caring God.

Whatever the reason, you may feel cut off from your church and from communication with God. You may go through a stage of change in which you lose your previous spiritual outlook and convictions. Not surprisingly, this loss brings with it strong feelings of anger, frustration, abandonment, and depression at a time when you already may be feeling alone and isolated from family and friends.

As they separate themselves from their religious convictions and their particular place of worship, some individuals block out any thoughts of God. Others question the beliefs and worldviews they've inherited, and then slowly find their way to their own, individual relationship with God, consciously developing a system of values they feel they can apply in good conscience to the circumstances and choices of their lives. Women who've been through this experience tell us they've learned that they can't control everything in their lives, that they now are able to think independently, and can order their lives according to their beliefs and not the beliefs of others. For them, the experience may lead to a deeper meaning of their spiritual purpose.

The Financial Burden

Adding to these emotional stresses is the major question of whether you can possibly afford the treatments that may bring you a child. If you live in any of the forty-three states that do not require insurance companies to pay for infertility treatments, the financial impact can be extreme. For example, gonadotropin hormones, commonly prescribed for stimulating egg development, can cost $2000 for each treatment cycle. In vitro fertilization costs anywhere from $7000 to $12,000 per cycle. For information on which states require infertility coverage, call RESOLVE (see page 235).

Looking Ahead

It is in these many ways that infertility can have an adverse effect on both your mental and physical well-being and on almost every aspect of your lives. If you've begun to stay away from family and friends, have no one to talk to about your feelings, feel abnormal because you don't have a child and are unable to talk about it with each other, it may be time to look for help. Unless you take steps early to avoid a possibly negative cycle of emotions, infertility can make your whole life turn sour.

The Connection Between Stress and Infertility

In recent years, a number of researchers, including those in our centers, have looked at the possible relationship between a variety of stressful emotions and infertility. Originally, many researchers interpreted stress to mean anxiety about being able to get pregnant. Using the standardized psychological measures for anxiety, they tested for this emotion as a possible factor in infertility. The results of the studies, however, turned out to be contradictory.

Some showed that anxiety had a detrimental effect on fertility and that a reduction in anxiety was tied to an increase in pregnancy rates. Other studies, however, found no relationship between the presence of anxiety and the rate of conception.

Beginning in the early 1990s, there was a shift away from viewing the psychological distress seen in infertile women as anxiety. Research began to be focused instead on the relationship between *depression* and infertility.

IS IT STRESS, ANXIETY, OR DEPRESSION?

Described here are the common symptoms of depression, anxiety, and stress.

Depression:

Feelings of inadequacy, hopelessness, sadness, and pessimism and a general loss of interest in life. Loss of appetite, difficulty sleeping, and lack of interest and enjoyment in your social activities and friends also are signs of depression. Other symptoms are a significant weight loss or gain or simply a change in appetite; tiredness most of the time; feelings of guilt and worthlessness; irritability and excessive anger over small things; difficulty concentrating; and decreases in effectiveness, activity, and productivity. Symptoms may get worse toward the end of the day and become more pronounced over time.

Anxiety:

This unpleasant emotional state ranges from mild uneasiness to intense fear and can include feelings of impending doom. These feelings should be taken seriously if they start to affect your thinking processes and disrupt your normal activities. Physical symptoms, such as heart palpitations, shortness of breath, hyperventilation, tense muscles in the back or neck, and gastrointestinal symptoms or discomfort, including vomiting, are common. Trembling and feeling shaky, having cold, sweaty palms, a dry mouth, flushes, chills, and the feeling of a lump in the throat are also symptoms. Others include feeling on edge, having your mind go blank, having trouble getting to sleep, and being irritable.

Stress:

This often is defined as any interference that disturbs a person's healthy mental and physical well-being. It can be a reaction to a wide range of physical and emotional stimuli, including internal/mental conflicts and significant life events. The body responds by increasing the production of certain hormones, including epinephrine and cortisol, as in the "fight or flight" response. Continued stress often leads to mental and physical symptoms such as *anxiety* and *depression,* heart palpitations, and muscle aches and pains.

We should point out, however, that the symptoms of anxiety, depression, and stress often can overlap and aren't necessarily clear-cut. When tested or interviewed by a mental health professional, persons who say they feel "distressed" or "stressed" might be diagnosed as being primarily depressed or primarily anxious. Furthermore, a lot of women and men might be depressed for years without realizing it until it gets in their way. Much research still needs to be done in this area, although at this point we and many others feel that, no matter what its formal label, psychological distress can have a negative effect on how the body functions, including its reproductive performance.

After a review of the studies that have been done on this question, the consensus of the investigators seems to be that anxiety may not play much of a role (although it has been associated with delayed conception in women preparing for donor insemination and an increased number of spontaneous abortions), but depression may contribute significantly to infertility.

In one study, for example, women with a history of depression were nearly twice as likely to experience infertility as women who didn't have such a history. In other research, women who already had several cycles of IVF treatment and were depressed before continuing it had a 13 percent pregnancy rate. Women who weren't depressed before receiving IVF had a 29 percent rate of conception.

Other research shows a clear relationship between depression and infertility. When a group of infertile women were compared to a matched control group of similar but fertile women, twice as many of the infertile women were found to be depressed, and a substantial proportion of them tested in the severe range.

Because a number of connections between depression and infertility have been made recently, our advice today is to examine your emotional/mental state carefully before you pursue infertility treatment.

If you have any reason to suspect you may be depressed, find professional help. Your physician, your HMO, friends who've had successful therapy for depression, or RESOLVE should be able to suggest where to find such therapy. The American Society for Reproductive Medicine has a Web site—www.asrm.org—that lists infertility counselors. You don't necessarily need a psychiatrist; other caregivers such as psychologists or social workers experienced with treating infertility-related depression can provide the help you may need. It can prove to be the best fertility enhancement you've tried. However, make sure you see someone who is well versed in the emotional impact of infertility.

IF YOU ARE TAKING ANTIDEPRESSANTS

If you know you're depressed and are taking antidepressants or other psychoactive drugs to treat it, it's important to continue. The weight of medical opinion today is that it is bet-

ter for a person who is clinically (seriously) depressed to remain on medication than to run the risk of another depressive
episode. There is no conclusive evidence that these drugs may
harm a fetus; however, they may affect your hormone levels. If
you aren't severely depressed, you will want to discuss with
your psychiatrist or a fertility endocrinologist the pros and
cons of remaining on this type of medication.

The Effect of Emotions on the Body

We're all aware of how anxiety or tension has an immediate effect
on our bodies. Our heart rate and breathing speed up and our
muscles tense, our stomach turns, we break out in a sweat. Our
bodies are alert and primed for action. This is the famous fight-
or-flight reaction that occurs when our brains perceive a threat.
Ordinarily this stress process stops when the perceived threat ends
and the brain then sets off certain calming changes within our
systems. However, if the worrying situation continues, or if the
brain doesn't recognize that it's ended, our stress reaction may
continue and become chronic, and our bodies don't calm down.

Harvard cardiologist Dr. Herbert Benson, the discoverer of the
well-known relaxation response, has pointed out that the human
fight-or-flight response and its countermeasure, the relaxation response, originate in the hypothalamus. The hypothalamus coor-
dinates the functions of the nervous and hormonal systems for
the entire body. It is connected to the nearby pituitary gland
through a short stalk of nerve fibers and controls the hormonal
secretions from this gland.

It occurred to us that there might be a connection between the
hypothalamic reaction to stress and the changes that take place in
hormone secretion. We also wondered if stress, often informally

linked to many ailments, could have a role in many of the disorders associated with the reproductive system. We wondered if stress-caused hormone imbalances might be a factor in menstrual irregularities, premenstrual syndrome (PMS), menopausal symptoms, infertility, and other problems associated with reproduction.

In the dozen years that have passed since we became intrigued by the possibility of such a connection, researchers here and at other institutions have shown that stress and a host of other negative emotions do indeed upset important, delicate hormonal balances in both women and men. Such imbalances can lead to irregular or missing menstrual cycles and may cause the fallopian tubes and uterus to contract and inhibit the movement of the egg into the uterus.

Stress and depression also have been implicated in the complete cessation of ovulation, called anovulatory amenorrhea. Furthermore, the production of excess adrenaline, one of the body's reactions to a fight-or-flight stimulus, in one study was linked to menstrual cycle irregularities. In men, emotional stress may be associated with abnormal sperm development.

Prolactin is a hormone released in large amounts by the pituitary gland when we are under a lot of physical stress—as in strenuous exercise—or emotional distress. High levels of prolactin in women lead to a lack of menstrual periods and infertility. In men, it may cause impotence.

GETTING HELP FOR INFERTILITY STRESS

Women who are tense and unhappy because they're having difficulty conceiving have a variety of resources from which to seek help: family, friends, professional therapists, RESOLVE, or other sources.

FAMILY OR FRIENDS. You may find your best help is your husband or partner. Or it can be a good friend, sibling, cousin, or acquaintance who has been through infertility herself. You'll want to make this choice with some care, seeking a person who is truly empathetic, who can be there for you over the long haul, in case it takes a while to resolve your infertility.

PROFESSIONAL HELP. You may wish to visit a professional who has expertise in the stresses of infertility. This could be a psychologist, social worker, psychiatrist, nurse therapist, or a religious counselor. The person's particular degree is not as important as her or his experience in dealing with the emotional side effects of not being able to become pregnant. The Web site of the American Society for Reproductive Medicine (www.asrm.org) is a good source for the names and locations of counselors who are members of the society and experienced in helping with these issues.

RESOLVE. You may want to turn to this organization, which was formed to help people cope with the experience of infertility. It has local chapters in every state that hold seminars, lectures, informal get-togethers, and helpful support groups usually led by professionals. The costs are relatively moderate. Chapters can refer patients to infertility specialists and to therapists. Furthermore, individual state chapters or RESOLVE's national office have information about the quality and success rates of infertility clinics nationwide. Many women feel that having a support group was the biggest help they had in getting their lives back.

RESOLVE is also a rich source for information on all aspects of the medical and emotional issues involved in infertility treatment, plus such alternatives as adoption and child-free living. It publishes a quarterly newsletter and fact sheets on more than fifty infertility-related subjects, ranging from anovulation to the zona-free hamster egg test.

RESOLVE is listed in the business section of the telephone book white pages. It is staffed almost entirely by volunteers who are familiar with the territory of infertility, infertility treatments, and the problems infertile couples can face, often from personal experience. In most cities, these volunteers spend evenings replying to calls left on the local chapter answering machine. If your community doesn't have a chapter, you can obtain information from RESOLVE's national office in Somerville, Massachusetts, at 617-623-0744.

THE HARVARD BEHAVIORAL MEDICINE PROGRAM FOR INFERTILITY

Behavioral or mind/body medicine teaches people to use their minds and bodies to change their behavior or their physiology in order to promote their health and/or recovery from illness. Behavioral medicine programs can be found by checking with the department of psychiatry, psychology, or medicine at your local hospital. Some HMOs may offer mind/body or stress management programs.

The behavioral medicine programs at the Beth Israel Deaconess Medical Center grew out of Dr. Herbert Benson's research and clinical work on the relaxation response and its ability to help people manage all sorts of difficult physiological conditions, including intractable chronic pain.

The infertility program is one of the behavioral medicine programs at Harvard that address women's disorders in particular. It grew out of our work on the relationships between stress, relaxation, and problems associated with the female reproductive system, including premenstrual syndrome, endometriosis, and menopause. The purpose of this program is to help women who are in a state of distress because of their infertility. In it we teach a variety of stress management strategies and relaxation techniques, and lead women to improve their overall health and well-being.

Since its very beginning the program has demonstrated that mind/body medicine can enable women with infertility to reclaim their lives and spirits. Our infertility program is now replicated in several other states in which there are affiliates of the Mind/Body Medical Institute. See page 234 in the Appendix for more information. The relaxation tapes we use are also listed (see pages 231–234).

Measuring the Effects of Stress Management

We began using behavioral medicine to help women manage the stress, depression, and other negative emotional fallout of infertility in 1987. From the very beginning we evaluated the women before and after they took part in the ten-session program. All had been seeing a physician for infertility. To measure their levels of depression and anxiety and other psychological symptoms, they were given a number of psychological tests before they began the program and after completing it. The first 106 women who completed the course demonstrated significant decreases in tension, anxiety, fatigue, and depression. They reported that they felt more vigorous and had increased feelings of control, security, well-being, and self-esteem. Furthermore, *34 percent of the first group of 54 women and 32 percent of the 52 women in the second group became pregnant within six months of completing the stress management program.*

Between 1989 and 1994 we evaluated a third group of 174 infertile women. Again, we used a battery of standard psychological questionnaires to measure their levels of depression and anxiety before and after they took part. A number of the women scored very high for depression (in the clinically depressed range) and for other problems, including physical complaints, hostility, and anxiety. When given at the end of the ten-session program, the same tests revealed that their negative emotions had dropped to the normal range.

These women had been struggling with infertility for one to ten years. Their average duration for infertility was more than three years and almost all were receiving medical treatment for it. Ages ranged from twenty-seven to forty-seven; the average age was thirty-five. The participants not only were able to reduce their levels of distress, but also *within six months of completing the program, 43.7 percent were pregnant.* Of these, just under 38 percent gave birth. We should point out, however, that the women who became pregnant tended to be younger than the women who did not conceive.

Of greatest interest to everyone involved in this particular study was the discovery that it was the women who were most stressed out, depressed, angry, and anxious who were most likely to conceive within six months. Sixty percent of those whose tests put them in the highest ranking for depression before they began the program became pregnant, compared to 24 percent of the women who were not depressed at all.

Startling as it may be, this finding makes sense to observers who are aware of the link between the emotions and the reproductive system. It seems entirely feasible that strong negative emotions can have a severe effect on the reproductive system. When this group of women learned to manage the distress of their infertility differently, their distress and its effects were substantially reduced and, in many cases, this allowed conception to occur. For those in the program who were not so upset, emotions may not have played a part in their infertility; instead, physical factors might have been the chief reason they couldn't conceive.

To explore further what we were seeing among the women attending the mind/body program, we decided to investigate formally the impact of different psychological interventions on infertility. To make the results as clear and definitive as possible, women of similar backgrounds, levels of depression, and infertility treatments would be randomly assigned to one of two psychological intervention groups *or* to a control group, in which women didn't participate in an intervention program. The two treatment groups would be modeled on those most available to women today: a support group like those offered by RESOLVE and a cognitive behavioral program similar to the one we offer at the Beth Israel Deaconess Medical Center. Members of the control group would continue with their lives and infertility treatments as usual.

THE STUDY

Our study became part of a large preventive intervention project on depression funded by the National Institute of Mental Health (NIMH). We examined whether an intervention could improve pregnancy rates in infertile women if it occurred early enough. Because this was a multicenter study, participants had to meet the requirement of the overall project—that they had tried to conceive for twelve to twenty-four months. Included where those with a history of miscarriage, who were single, had secondary infertility, or had poor infertility treatment prospects, such as having high FSH levels or many treatment failures. Those who couldn't be included were women who had been trying to become pregnant for more than two years. In addition, women who were found to be clinically depressed by the psychological tests were referred elsewhere for treatment and were not accepted for the study.

As women entered the study they were assigned at random into one of the three groups: control, support, and cognitive behavioral (or mind/body). There were no differences among the groups in the percentage of women receiving infertility treatments, nor were there any differences in the types of medical treatments.

Women who signed on agreed to be followed as part of our research for four years, which meant that they could not seek another type of psychological intervention or, if they were in the control group, *any* psychological treatment for that span of time. Women were not discouraged from seeking such assistance, but if they did, they could no longer participate in the study.

In addition, a psychologist who didn't know which woman was in what group administered a series of psychological tests to each participant twice a year for the four-year period, to evaluate her level of distress. Each woman also was asked to record her fertility medications and treatments on a monthly basis. And women in the support and control groups were asked not to start any type of relaxation practice, including yoga, for the four years of the study, so that they would remain different from the members of the cognitive behavioral groups, who did practice relaxation techniques. Participants were to contact researchers if they conceived. The primary outcome measurement of the study was a live birth.

The format of the two interventions—support and cognitive behavioral—was identical, but the content of their sessions differed. Both met once a week for ten weeks for two hours in the evening.

Cognitive Behavioral Segment

Women in the cognitive behavioral groups learned ways to elicit the relaxation response and many coping skills. They also were given information on nutrition and exercise that was relevant to fertility, such as stopping exercise and cutting back on caffeine. Although the content of this intervention resembled in many ways the infertility program we've offered since 1987, a number of its aspects weren't included. Husbands didn't attend any sessions, there was no sharing period at the beginning of each meeting, and each session was exactly two hours long. These modifications made the format of the two types of interventions the same.

Support Segment

The support groups spent the first hour of each session checking in with one another, discussing personal issues, and finding out how each member was feeling. The second hour was spent on a discussion topic, different each week, such as the impact of infertility on self-esteem, relationships with partners or friends, and the effect of infertility events on their jobs or careers.

Control Group

The women assigned to this group received no intervention at all, but simply continued with their regular infertility treatments. The types of treatments they were using were very much the same as those used by the women in the intervention groups. No group was weighted toward one type or degree of treatment.

In the beginning, 56 women participated in the cognitive behavioral intervention groups, 65 took part in support groups, and 63 were in the control group. However, 38 of the 63 women in the control segment bowed out of the study before the end of its first year because they were too depressed to go without psychological treatment. (They did not know about the pregnancies occurring in the other groups.) Most of them joined a RESOLVE support group or a clinical behavioral program. As a result, only 25 control group participants could be followed for the entire first year. There also were some dropouts from the intervention groups: by the end of the first year, 48 of the women who participated in support groups and 47 who were in the cognitive behavioral groups remained in the study.

The Results

Within twelve months of entering the study, *55 percent of the* women in the cognitive behavioral group and *54 percent in the support group had conceived pregnancies that resulted in live births.* Of the 25 women who remained in the control group, however, 5 had viable pregnancies, a viable pregnancy rate of 20 percent, barely over one-third of the rate of those in the psychological intervention groups.

The women underwent their second session of psychological testing six months after they had been assigned to one of the three groups. It was found that those in the two intervention groups experienced more positive changes in self-actualization (how they saw themselves in the context of their world), interpersonal support, use of stress management skills, episodes of anxiety, and marital distress than did the women in the control group. They also showed a trend toward less depression.

On all the psychological measurements, however, the women in the control group revealed that their symptoms were worsening, while those in the two intervention groups showed a moderate improvement in symptoms. The cognitive behavioral group experienced the most improvement in psychological symptoms.

The difference in pregnancy rates was not due to any differences in the women's backgrounds, including their age and the length of their infertility. Nor was it due to differences in medical treatments among the groups. The same percentage of women in each group pursued the various types of medical assistance currently available, including the newer technologies.

This research underscores what has been seen in other infertile women who sought psychological assistance to relieve their symptoms of depression—that alleviating depression and other psychological distress appears to make it easier to become pregnant. And it appears that the form of an intervention may not be as important as the fact that, whatever it is, it mitigates the distress.

Thanks to other research we know that psychological distress has an impact on many body systems, including inhibiting the secretion of the hormones necessary for reproduction. Changes in hormone levels, in turn, can affect ovulation, fertilization of the egg, the function of the fallopian tubes, and the readiness of the uterus to accept an embryo.

Whether or not women who have been infertile for longer than two years would also benefit from some sort of psychological assistance remains to be studied; our experience at the Division of Behavioral Medicine of the Beth Israel Deaconess Medical Center for the past dozen years indicates that women with long-term infertility may well increase their chances of conception when they reduce their levels of depression. It may even be sensible for women who want to get pregnant and suspect they are depressed to treat such depression first, before trying to conceive.

We'd like to point out again that it appears that the exact content of the intervention may not be as important as how effective it is at relieving depression. Other studies clearly show that women achieve psychological benefit from attending programs that are somewhat different yet similar to the ones we used in this research. We feel that such programs should be offered at an earlier step in the treatment staircase—perhaps before women start their first medical treatments.

The cost of psychological intervention groups ranges from $100 to $800. Some insurance plans may cover this type of treatment. Becoming a member of a RESOLVE support group is probably the least expensive approach, and that organization has support groups in almost all localities. To find other sources of help in your area, see those included in "Organizations That Can Help" in the Appendix, pages 235–238. If none are listed for where you live, check with the nearest infertility clinics or a reproductive medical specialist (and their nursing staffs) for suggestions on where to find psychological assistance.

FOLLOWING THE HARVARD PROGRAM AT HOME

With the help of some additional reading (see our reading list, page 238), it's also possible to follow our program for infertile women without joining a group. We often teach the same methods to individuals in one-on-one sessions. The only missing element would be the group connections and sharing. These are important, and it may be possible to cultivate them by joining a RESOLVE support group or by forming your own group with other infertile women (your doctor or nurse may be able to help you do this). A group doesn't have to be large to be supportive. If forming a group isn't feasible, you simply may want to find at least one other like-minded, infertile woman who can get together with you once a week. Besides sharing feelings and comparing notes about infertility incidents, you can help each other learn the relaxation techniques and other exercises described in this chapter.

The Program Structure

As we noted, the program consists of ten sessions. There are eight regular sessions of two and one-half hours, plus one half-day and one all-day session. Husbands attend the first, seventh, and ninth sessions. Each gathering is preceded by an optional half-hour period of sharing and support time that gives the women a chance to talk among themselves, to share their infertility experiences and what they're learning about coping. This time together encourages the group to form bonds and begin to function also as a support group. Each group has about sixteen members on average.

At the first session, participants are introduced to one another and then paired off with a buddy, a woman who lives near her. Buddies telephone each other at least once a week and each buddy pair takes a turn bringing a snack for the whole group. (Learning about the importance of *healthy* snacking is part of the program—except, of course, when we encourage the group to have something chocolate for dessert!) We then introduce the participants to the dynamics of the fight-or-flight response—its physiology and its physical/psychological consequences—and how the relaxation response counters the effects of such consequences. Participants are given their first lesson on how to elicit the relaxation response.

We introduce the relaxation response at our first session and guide participants as they practice it. At each subsequent session we teach other ways to achieve the response and give members plenty of time to practice it. Through your reading or by finding a class in meditation or yoga you can learn these techniques on your own. What's important—what makes the relaxation response effective—is using it every day.

Session I: The Relaxation Response

We recommend at our first session that some form of relaxation be practiced daily for about twenty minutes. If you are especially stressed, you may want to elicit the relaxation response twice a day. Other than that recommendation, for the successful practice of the relaxation response you chiefly need to be aware of your own needs and lifestyle. You may want to experiment with various approaches before finding the relaxation method or methods that are effective for you. What probably is most important as you build the relaxation response into your daily life is finding a ritual that works and is a good fit for you. If you can't find the time every day, don't feel guilty. Just keep coming back to it. Your relaxation exercise eventually will feel so good that you will miss it when you can't do it.

THE RELAXATION RESPONSE

The relaxation response was discovered in the late 1960s by Harvard cardiologist Dr. Herbert Benson, when he learned that the practice of transcendental meditation had remarkable physical and psychological effects on those who used it. He also found that these effects could be evoked by many different relaxation methods, and he named the changes that occurred the relaxation response. Dr. Benson's research led him to theorize that this reaction was a natural, built-in mechanism designed to counteract the effects of our automatic fight-or-flight response.

The relaxation response is actually a series of changes that take place in the body and mind as they grow calm. A number of techniques can be used to evoke the response, including yoga, repetitive prayer, deep breathing, meditation, progressive muscle relaxation, and visual imagery. Regardless of what method is used, the physiologic changes are the same: heart rate, muscle tension, breathing rate, and oxygen consumption fall below resting levels. Normal waking brain waves change to distinctive, usually slower patterns.

As you can see, this isn't simply learning to "relax." By regularly eliciting the relaxation response, individuals are able to lower their blood pressure and their heart and breathing rates. The relaxation response also has been successful in reducing the pain of such physical disorders as endometriosis, rheumatoid arthritis, chronic fatigue syndrome, fibromyalgia, menstrual cramps, and headaches, including migraines. Its regular use helps reduce the side effects of chemotherapy and can ease the symptoms of irritable bowel syndrome and anxiety disorders. In the infertility program, relaxation training is used to reduce physical symptoms such as insomnia and psychological problems like anxiety.

For the woman with infertility, practicing relaxation can be both body and mind altering. One of the depressing aspects of infertility is that you feel you have no control over your body. It isn't doing what you always assumed it would and may not react to treatments designed to make it respond. And unsuccessful cycles of fertility treatments can make you feel even more helpless. When you begin regularly practicing a relaxation exercise, you may realize for the first time just how tense you are and how angry you are—at your body, your husband, your family, for not understanding; at medical personnel who may be less than compassionate. This is when you can acknowledge how much you've been enduring and consciously begin the process of healing.

You will need to put aside the idea that you are doing this in order to conceive. If you continue to stay focused on pregnancy, it's likely you may not truly relax. Your purpose in undertaking a program like this is to get your life back. For meditation, we've found that one of the most powerful—and appropriate—mantras, or focus phrases, is "Let go." This does not imply that you should give up; it simply means that you are dropping from your mind and body all the tension and anxiety of infertility.

Session II: More Relaxation Techniques

There are many methods you can use to achieve the relaxation response: breath focus (also called diaphragmatic breathing), body scan, progressive muscle relaxation, meditation, prayer, mindfulness, guided imagery, autogenic training, yoga, or any relaxation ritual you develop for yourself. Descriptions of the practice of these can be found in a number of books, including *Healing Mind, Healthy Woman,* by Dr. Alice Domar and Henry Dreher (New York: Dell, 1997).

One relaxation technique is guided imagery, which often is used to diminish the side effects of chemotherapy and reduce pain in cancer patients. It's also a powerful method for improving your quality of life because it brings you to a deep peacefulness. You can use an audiotape to help you through a particular exercise in imagery, or you can develop your own imagery.

✦ Practicing Guided Imagery:

1. Sit comfortably in a quiet place.
2. Take several slow, deep breaths.
3. Now picture in your mind's eye a place that you love, a place where you have been relaxed or you feel you could be relaxed.
4. Visualize yourself strolling or sitting or standing within this scene, slowly absorbing its views, sounds, and lovely fragrances.
5. If the scene is outdoors, take in the color of the sky and the shape of the clouds. Look at the green of the trees and grass. If it's a beach, notice the pattern that waves leave in the sand or the tranquility of a lake's gentle motion. Watch the birds circling high above.
6. Now concentrate on the smells: If you're in a meadow, inhale the scent of sun-warmed grass. If it's a woods, breathe in deeply the fragrance of moist leaves. Smell the salty, fishy air of the ocean beach or the special rainwater aroma of the lake.
7. Focus on sounds indoors or outside: the chitter-chatter of a squirrel, the song of a robin or blackbird, the slap of waves

against the side of a boat, children playing, soft music, rain falling against the windows.

8. Concentrate on sensations: the warmth of the sun on your back or rain on your face. If you see yourself walking bare-footed across a sun-dappled lawn, feel the tickle of the grass on your feet. Or, if it's a beach, how the damp sand moves beneath your feet.

9. Let yourself sink into the sensual aspects of your images. Relish your comfort, your pleasure, your tranquility. If you're disturbed by anxious thoughts, look at them for a minute, then gently return to the sights, scents, and sensations that surround you.

If you find it difficult to take yourself to an imaginary place, don't feel troubled. Not everyone can do this readily. Instead, try to find a method that might help transport you. We sometimes suggest that you imagine yourself on a magic carpet that carries you to your peaceful place. Or visualize yourself floating away on your own, like the children in *Peter Pan,* off to your very own Never-Never Land.

Learning about a variety of relaxation techniques enables the participants of the program and anyone learning this at home to find at least one that works well for them. Or you may discover that combining several is more effective than using just one. As long as it works, tailor your routine to suit you—using it regularly is the key. The audiotapes we've listed in the Appendix (pages 231–234) may help.

PRACTICING MINI-RELAXATIONS. In addition to regular relaxation techniques, it can be very useful to learn mini-relaxation exercises. Minis are shorter—brief exercises of diaphragmatic breathing that switch a person to deep, slow breathing from the hasty, shallow breathing we all use when we're upset or anxious. Shallow breathing doesn't allow enough oxygen to reach our brains and bodies, thus aggravating the fight-or-flight response, keeping us tense and often making us breathe even harder. The great advantage of minis is that they can be done quickly, any-where and anytime you feel anxious or anticipate feeling anxious. You can do them with other people around without anyone sus-pecting that you're practicing a relaxation technique. They're highly useful to calm yourself before an IVF procedure, or before asking your boss for time off (or a raise), or when you're anxious about anything. We teach participants in the behavioral medicine programs four versions—all equally quick and helpful. They also are outlined in *Healing Mind, Healthy Woman.*

᷐ Mini-version 1:

1. Sit down or lie down in a comfortable position.
2. Take a *deep, slow* breath. Notice any movement in your chest or abdomen.
3. Place a hand on your abdomen, just over your belly button, and allow your abdomen to rise about an inch as you inhale.
4. Then, as you exhale, notice that your abdomen will fall about an inch. Also notice that your chest rises slightly with your ab-domen. (Abdominal breathing doesn't mean that you don't bring air into your upper chest; you do. But now you are also bringing air down into the lower part of your lungs by using your diaphragm to expand the entire chest cavity.)
5. Become aware of your diaphragm moving down as you inhale and up as you exhale. Remember that it's impossible to breathe abdominally if your diaphragm doesn't move down. And it's impossible to let your diaphragm move down if your stomach muscles are tight. So relax your stomach muscles! If this is difficult, try breathing in through your nose and out through your mouth. Enjoy the sensations of abdominal breathing for several breaths or for as long as you want.

✦ *Mini-version 2:*

1. Make the shift from chest breathing to deep abdominal breathing.
2. Count down from ten to zero, taking one complete breath—one inhale, one exhale—with each number. Thus, with your first abdominal breath, you say ten to yourself, with the next breath you say nine, and so on. If you start to feel light-headed or dizzy, slow down your count. When you reach zero, see how you're feeling. If you're feeling more relaxed, excellent! If not, try doing it again.

✦ *Mini-version 3:*

1. Make the shift from chest breathing to deep abdominal breathing.
2. As you inhale, count very slowly from one to four.
3. As you exhale, count slowly from four to one. This means you are silently saying to yourself as you inhale, one, two, three, four. And as you exhale you think, four, three, two, one. Do this at least several times, or longer if you wish.

✦ *Mini-version 4:*

1. Make the shift to abdominal breathing, using any of these methods.
2. This time, regardless of which method you're using, pause for a few seconds after each in-breath and again after each out-breath. Do this at least several times—or longer.

As we've said, minis can be done in a variety of everyday circumstances when you need to catch your tension on the rise and stop it. Minis are helpful in a lot of situations; women we know use them during a blood test, before making one of those important telephone calls, during a pelvic exam or ultrasound, or before giving themselves an injection. You can do them in a waiting room or while stuck in traffic—they take only a few minutes and perform wonders. The simple process of breathing can be an immediate source of relaxation and control if you use it this way.

Session III: Be Good to Yourself

Session III of the infertility mind/body program is focused on teaching the participants how to be good to themselves, which is another way of saying they learn to tend to their needs. Women are notorious for ignoring their own needs and wishes in favor of putting their husbands or partners first. They see their role as being the nurturing person among their families and friends. Women with low self-esteem particularly are more comfortable as givers than receivers of care and attention. Unfortunately, constantly denying her own feelings and desires, swallowing the irritation and anger that are inevitable in anyone's life, and always being the one who's there in a pinch uses up a woman's emotional and physical reserves. Eventually it becomes detrimental to her mental and physical health. Just as we have taught women to discover what interests and pleases them and how to build some pleasure into each day of their lives in order to replenish themselves, you can learn to do this for yourself.

PLEASURE IS GOOD FOR YOUR HEALTH

In scientific studies, pleasures, particularly those that involve our senses, have been seen to enhance not only our feeling of well-being but our health as well. The studies suggest that our nervous, cardiovascular, and immune systems respond as positively to sensual experiences as do our minds. For example, gazing at an attractive aquarium of handsome tropical fish was found not only to be relaxing but it lowered blood pressure levels as well. An empty tank didn't have the same effect. Music, pleasant aromas, and the tastes of certain foods also have been used successfully to relax people and to reduce pain, depression, and stress.

Before you can build pleasure into your life, however, you need to realize that it's vital to your health. You also need to feel you are worthwhile enough as a person to make time in your life for your own enjoyment. This isn't only a self-esteem issue. Putting yourself last is part of the identity of most females, handed down from preceding generations of women. The stressed-out, anxious woman of today, however, who wants to improve her mental and physical health, needs to rethink this old model and give herself permission to nurture herself and have some fun. For additional help on this subject, see Dr. Domar's book *Self-Nurture* (Viking, 2000).

WHAT PLEASES *YOU?*

Think hard! What would give you the most pleasure? It doesn't have to be something major or expensive—you can treat yourself to a bunch of flowers, a manicure, a new mystery novel. Have a long soak in the tub, preferably with a wonderful bath oil or aromatherapy scent. Window-shop. Find someone to clean your house and—most important—spend the time that's saved on yourself. Get together with women whose lives are not centered on children. Go canoeing with your husband. Join a book club. Build more movies into your life. Spend a weekend together in the country and forget what time of month it is. Whatever you enjoy, think of it as a doctor's prescription for your mental health and do it regularly.

PRACTICING PLEASURE. Now that you have some ideas of how to be good to yourself, take a piece of paper and write down all the wonderful things you'd like to do or have someone do for you. What gives you real pleasure? Or joy?

- Reading the Sunday papers outdoors with a glass of freshly made fruit juice or a mug of hot chocolate.
- Buying something you don't need but really want.
- Treating yourself to a haircut at one of the best salons.
- Not going to your in-laws for the next holiday.
- Playing hooky once every few months from your job.
- Choosing a lot of unusual new plants for your home.
- Lounging in a comfortable chair and reading a mystery.
- Taking naps as often as possible.
- Walking in a different part of town or in the country each week.
- Planting an herb garden or sweet-scented flowers indoors or near your back door.
- Taking your husband out for lunch somewhere new.

We often ask the women in our program to draw a circle on a sheet of paper and divide it, pie-like, into segments that represent their average day, including time for sleeping, commuting, work, running errands, and watching TV. Try this at home. Label each slice with the activity and number of hours or minutes you spend on it. Be as accurate as possible.

One Woman's 24-hour Time Pie

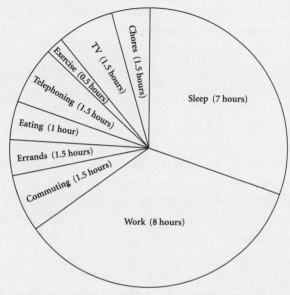

Next, take your list of all the pastimes and activities that give you pleasure. How many of them are included in your time pie? If you did a chart of a typical week in your life, how many pleasures or joys would you see there? Can they be measured in hours—or only in minutes?

If you are serious about the importance of nurturing yourself and changing your approach to life, take your daily time pie and reconfigure it. Create more time for the most important enjoyments on your list. Be realistic—you want this to work, don't you? Look particularly for the areas where you spend time trying to relax but don't really, such as collapsing in front of the TV or chatting on the phone. Lots of trips for groceries? Order them for delivery, instead. It will focus your menu planning into a single list for the week—and give you several hours to spend on something that renews your spirit. Now work some fun and joy into your time pie. A daily half hour or one hour several times a week of doing something you relish is as important to your health as any medicine a doctor might prescribe.

Session IV: Exercise, Yoga, Mindfulness

The fourth session is four and a half hours from early evening on, and begins with the participants being taught the principles and practice of hatha yoga. It is followed by a healthful but yummy dinner and a talk about the effects of nutrition and exercise on fertility. The impact of either too much or too little weight is covered, much along the lines discussed in Step 1. And participants learn about a different approach to exercise for infertile women.

WHEN YOU SHOULDN'T EXERCISE. In most relaxation courses designed to manage other physical problems, regular exercise is encouraged as a good way to relax. For infertile women, however, we have different advice. Those women who have no chance of getting pregnant spontaneously because their infertility is caused by totally blocked fallopian tubes, or by a severe male factor, are told to stop exercising completely during those cycles when they are receiving injectable medicines, such as in IVF. During monthly cycles when they are not being treated, they can continue their regular exercise patterns.

Infertile women who may conceive spontaneously are advised to stop exercising entirely for three months or at least to indulge in *only very mild exercises* that will not raise their heart rate over 110 beats. They must stroll instead of walking briskly and can continue with any yoga or stretching exercises. They should not undertake anything vigorous or aerobic, in order to see if exercise is having an adverse effect on their ability to conceive. This is a good time for slow, mindful walks (less than two miles!) with their partners or friends.

If they are not pregnant within three months, however, we tell them that they can assume exercise was not a problem and they can go back to their usual athletic regimens—if they're moderate. We realize this advice may sound odd because exercise is so good for people, but the fact is that we've seen an extraordinary number of pregnancies in women who stopped exercising for a short time.

It's important to note, however, that if you are stressed and you stop exercising, your anxiety levels quite likely will rise. Therefore, as you stop exercising, it's an especially good idea to start practicing the relaxation response, or any other stress management technique that works for you, to help you handle negative emotions.

PRACTICING YOGA. This is a particularly good method of relaxing and using your body in a nonstressful way. Hatha yoga is the form we teach in our program. It doesn't require pretzel-like positions; instead, it can be done while sitting in a chair or on the floor, or standing. Hatha yoga combines breathing exercises with slow, gentle movements and postures that stretch the body and release tensions.

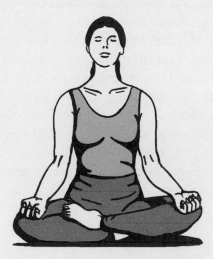

It's possible to learn yoga from books, but it has been our experience that it's best learned from a teacher, if you can find a class in your community. If you have a choice of classes, select an instructor who inspires your commitment and will give you advice on postures and adjustments suited to your body. If you can't find a class or want to learn more about yoga, the books we recommend include *Yoga for Women,* by Paddy O'Brien (New York: Harper Collins, 1995), and *Complete Stretching Book,* by Maxine Tobias (New York: Random House, 1992). In *The Wellness Book* (New York: Fireside, 1992), by Dr. Herbert Benson, Eileen Stuart, and the staff of The Mind/Body Medical Institute, there's a chapter, "Tuning In to Your Body, Tuning Up Your Mind," by Margaret Ennis, in which she offers a variety of yoga exercise with clear directions.

Yoga is particularly good for women whose minds are so full of what they have to do they can't turn them off long enough to focus on eliciting the relaxation response. By releasing muscle tension, yoga helps to quiet the mind. Yoga also appears to have spiritual and psychological benefits for women who are struggling with infertility. It can help you to experience yourself as someone who is whole and complete.

PRACTICING MINDFULNESS. At this same dinner session the group also learns about the practice of mindfulness. Mindfulness teaches us to live in the here and now and to enjoy the sensations of our bodies and our senses right at this moment. One of the peculiar effects of infertility is that it tends to be so totally absorbing. Your concentration is on what the next step in the treatment process is, on what your ovulation test will show tomorrow, whether you dare go on that business trip next month, did you have sex often enough last month, and so on. Soon there is no room in your mind for what is actually going on around you right now.

By being mindful, by concentrating on every aspect of something you're doing, such as eating an ice cream cone, walking slowly through a quiet art museum, choosing plants from a tropical greenhouse, or even learning an absorbing new skill, you are both relaxing and nurturing yourself. Your feelings of being stressed out can vanish as you focus on finding pleasure in this particular moment. What activity you choose doesn't matter—what counts is your awareness as you go about it.

Here's one example of a mindful activity:

1. Take an orange in your hand and notice the texture of its skin and the way it feels and smells.
2. Peel it slowly. Notice the fragrance of citrus as you unhurriedly pull off each piece of peel.
3. Then gently tear each segment apart. Notice the symmetry.
4. As you bite into each one, pay attention to the ooze of juice, the tang of the citrus in your mouth and nostrils.
5. Eat slowly and savor every taste, including the last bit of juice that you lick from your fingers.

Remember that the purpose of mindfulness is the deliberate cultivation of your awareness of the here and now. You can enjoy an entire meal, wash vegetables, fold clothes, make love, or take a walk mindfully. The key is to slow down and engage all your senses in what you are doing.

IF YOUR MIND WANDERS

As you practice a relaxation technique or mindfulness, don't be disturbed if thoughts of other things intrude. Jon Kabat-Zinn, of the Stress Reduction Clinic at the University of Massachusetts Medical Center, says: "If you have a mind, it is going to wander." It's important that you accept this tendency rather than scold yourself for it. It's a natural process. Learn to watch each thought as it comes and goes. Be mindful of your process of thinking. Notice how thoughts shift, move, dissolve. If you lose track of what you're trying to do, don't get upset. Simply observe what is happening. If you're doing a relaxation exercise, return gently to being aware of your breath. Try to keep breathing in the forefront of your mind and allow your thoughts and other distractions to continue in the background. Don't fight such thoughts, just be aware of them, and return to your breathing.

Sessions V and VI: Cognitive Restructuring

The next two sessions are devoted to revealing just how nasty are the thoughts of the woman who is infertile—and how to challenge and restructure them. Women in general are susceptible to negative thoughts, most of them the legacy of our culture and our families. Quite a few of these thoughts have to do with mistakes we've made or think we've made, or how we're not normal and have no value if we don't have children. There are voices in our heads that say we don't deserve to have children or that we won't be good mothers. When we don't conceive as soon as we expected to, these thoughts come surging to the forefront of our minds, running over and over again like a tape loop: I don't deserve to have a child. Why did I wait? If only I had tried to get pregnant sooner. I can't do anything right.

All of us have negative tape loops in our heads and some of them can be downright defeating. They're especially harmful when you're struggling with infertility and already fear failure because these silent voices can really contribute to depression and stress. Women in the mind/body programs are taught how to uncover such messages, and to check to see where these thoughts come from and if they're valid. They also are coached in how to discover the reality of their situations and to replace their nasty mental tapes with more truthful and compassionate messages.

This skill, called cognitive restructuring, is described further in *Healing Mind, Healthy Woman* and in *Self-Nurture*.

PRACTICING COGNITIVE RESTRUCTURING. Without thinking about it too much, quickly write down the most common tapes that run through your mind. Whose voice are you hearing? Your mother's or father's? A brother's or sister's? Your critical aunt's? A coach's you could never please?

The basic exercise for changing any negative mental tape that you identify requires that you ask yourself four questions about it:

1. Does this thought contribute to my stress?
2. Where did I learn this thought?
3. Is this thought logical?
4. Is this thought true?

The purpose of these questions is to confront that thought honestly, figure out its source and look at its effect on you, and then put it to the test of logic. If you can't determine by yourself whether a nasty recurring thought is logical or true, you may need the help of a friend who can be fair and analytical and whose judgment you trust. Apply your intelligence, self-awareness, and honesty with precision and you will discover surprising truths about your automatic thoughts and their effect on your state of mind and health. Be rigorous about this. You may also discover that the opposite of your negative thoughts is what is *really* true about you.

The thought we hear most often in the program is "I'll never have a baby," which is not surprising coming from women who've been trying to have a child for years. Nevertheless, we ask them to be more tough-minded when they contemplate that tape. This is a typical dialogue with a participant (try it with yourself):

Q. Is this thought contributing to your stress?
A. Absolutely.
Q. Where did you learn this thought?

A. I'm not sure.

Q. Did your doctor say you could not have a biological child?

A. No, he never said that. He thinks I could have one.

Q. Is your thought logical?

A. I guess not. As far as I know, I can still have a biological child.

Q. Is your thought true?

A. I can't say that. It may or may not be. No one can predict the future.

Q. Why do you continue to get treatment for infertility?

A. So I can have a baby!

Q. Then part of you must believe it is possible, or why would you continue to expend so much time and energy?

A. I guess part of me does think it's possible.

The honest restructuring of this particular—and common—negative thought becomes "I could have a baby." This lies somewhere between the totally negative, frightening thought, "I'll never have a baby," and the Pollyanna statement, "Of course I'll have a baby." It's a more realistic and honest thought that often can lift a woman's spirit as she pursues her path through treatments for infertility.

VANESSA'S STORY

When I discovered that intrauterine insemination wouldn't work for me and I'd have to use in vitro fertilization, I was really scared. I had been told that IVF was my "last option." I was already under a lot of stress because of my job and because of the infertility process and this was the last straw. I was so upset.

What I've learned in the mind/body program has helped me, but it's been hard to recognize that I'm more than just an infertile woman, that infertility is just one part of my life. I was so fixated on my cycle. Now I'm trying to realize that infertility is not the center of my universe. I'm making time for the relaxation exercise. It really helps calm me down.

I'm discovering that we have a lot more options than I thought—there's the egg donor program and there's adoption. And I've learned not to be frightened away from these options because of the scare stories in the media.

When my fears of never becoming a mother crowd into my mind, I use cognitive restructuring to push them out. I just say to myself, Does this thought help you at all? Can you do something about this or are you just worrying? So, until I can get more facts, I just put that thought away. Then I get really busy doing something else. I find that it helps to try to catch negative thoughts early.

Sessions VII and VIII: Expressing Emotions

The next coping skill the program teaches is how to express painful emotions fully—and without actually blasting the persons causing the pain. Not surprisingly, anger is usually one of the strongest feelings an infertile woman has. She is likely to be angry at her body for betraying her, angry at her husband for not understanding, and angry at doctors and other medical staff for putting her through so much unpleasantness and then perhaps not showing compassion when she needs it.

PRACTICING JOURNALING. What we tell women is that if you are angry, write down exactly how you feel and why. Get it all out because if you don't get to the very bottom of your feelings, you may feel worse. Start keeping a journal and keep going back to it—even for only ten minutes a day.

Bringing out your feelings will help you unbury events and emotions you may have experienced years ago that are affecting you now. Putting it down on paper will help you come to terms with much of the negative burden you may not even realize you are carrying. And don't limit yourself to your angry feelings—use your journal to write down all your feelings: your grief, anxiety, hopes, weariness, disgust, despair, humor, and self-discovery. You may gain fresh insights into your emotions and your stress. The writing, like the relaxation exercise, eventually may help you think more clearly about your issues.

Husbands/partners are invited to the seventh session. They meet with a male psychologist to share their feelings about infertility and the impact it's having on them. At all three sessions that include spouses, the men discover that this program is not an all-female kaffee klatsch of complaints. They learn how to elicit the relaxation response themselves, they and their spouses hear a talk about the ins and outs of adoption, and during the all-day Sunday meeting, they practice yoga together.

If you're practicing self-care at home and want to include your partner, and he's willing, you can teach him one—or several—of your relaxation exercises. He not only will have a better idea of what you're doing, but he may find the exercise useful in his life as well.

Session IX: Paired Listening Exercise

Another couples exercise that builds on this can also be done at home. In the ninth session of the program, couples are given private spaces. Then each partner takes a turn at talking while the other listens. They speak about three subjects: something they like about their spouse that they've never mentioned, something they like about themselves that they've never told, and something they like about their relationship that they never said. After this, we see couples returning to the group who are absolutely glowing with a sense of well-being.

Such exercises in communication between couples are designed to heal cracks in marriages that may have developed during years of struggling with infertility. Women and men seldom share the same view of where they are going with infertility—how far to go with treatments, for instance, or whether adoption could be an option for them. It can be extremely useful to work on understanding each other early in the struggle. This not only is an exercise for when you're infertile; it also may benefit your relationship if you continue to practice it regularly throughout your married life.

WYNN'S STORY

Being infertile is ridiculously awful. Everything bothers me—I'm up and then I'm down. After each shot I feel a little bit optimistic until I ovulate and then I start feeling really negative. I feel that I'm not pregnant and then I just feel I'm about to have my period. There's such a sense of dread.

Lately there've been a lot of babies born to people where I work. My boss's wife had a baby and he's been complaining a lot about how hard it's made their life. I could just kill him. Then he brought the baby in last week and the little guy was just so cute—I went home and cried.

In a way, my husband and I have found that our lives have been enriched by working through this experience. We feel so solid as a couple, and I think we wouldn't have known this feeling without going through infertility. Now we're even able—finally—to joke about the angry feelings I have that could come out in some of our social situations. Today, when I see a pregnant woman, I'll say something like "infertile woman goes berserk," and then we break up laughing.

Session X: How to Say No

In the last session of the program, participants learn how to say no without feeling guilty, in an exercise we learned from Dr. Matthew Budd. Members go off in pairs, and then one person in each pair goes through a list of requests that would be hard to turn down, such as: Can I borrow a quarter for a phone call? Will you please move closer so I can hear you better? Will you come to my house for dinner? The other half of the pair must say no to each of these pleasant requests.

Questioners are then told to keep pursuing their requests and respondents are told to make up any kind of reason for saying no. The women learn to be nimble in coming up with good reasons for turning down even reasonable requests.

This exercise teaches three different ways to turn down requests: a simple no; no, but how about such and such; and no, because . . . and give a reason. Participants practice using these responses because they provide ways for women—who often are too inclined to say yes—to protect themselves from situations that infringe on their boundaries and energy reserves. To quote psychologist colleague Ann Webster: "Sometimes to say no to someone else is to say yes to ourselves."

Also during this session a short list of categories is handed out to the participants. The list includes health, relationships, career-job-volunteer work, spirituality, creativity, material objects, and play. They are asked to close their eyes, take several deep, relaxing breaths, and describe where they want to be in their lives three months from now. The women write down these goals as a letter to themselves and address it. The letters are mailed to them three months later so that they can see how they're progressing.

To end this last session, participants close their eyes and view what they've learned in the program as a mountain they've climbed to the very top—and relish the vista that now stretches ahead of them.

These exercises can be practiced at home. You not only can rehearse the ways to say no, but also you can teach yourself to recognize when it's important and appropriate to turn down a request. And the exercise of writing down the categories of goals, closing your eyes, breathing deeply, and visualizing what you'd like to do in those categories will help you set your goals. Write them down and stick them in your calendar to look at three months from now. Close your eyes, climb your mountain, and see what your life may hold for you.

ACQUIRING THE HABIT OF STRESS MANAGEMENT

If you're just beginning the infertility experience, the mind/body exercises and skills we've been describing can be incorporated into your life early on to avoid many of infertility's tensions and distresses. If you want to protect your marriage and the well-being of your partner and yourself, we suggest the following:

- Nurture yourself and your health with behavioral medicine, particularly the relaxation techniques. If your partner seems interested, encourage him (or her) to join you in such self-care.
- Use the communication exercises just described to keep yourself open to each other. Share your efforts at self-care with your partner, but do so without accusations or defensiveness.
- Find or form a support group of women who also are experiencing infertility. Get in touch with RESOLVE and use its resources for support groups and information.
- Use the Internet—carefully—to collect information on infertility and its many treatments and to locate or form a woman's support group if there's no RESOLVE chapter in your town. There is a great deal of information on all aspects of infertility on the Internet. Use any of the popular search engines to look under "health" and "reproductive health," as well as "infertility." *Bear in mind, however, that the medical information you find on the Internet can be inaccurate or may not be the answer for your particular problem.* It's best to use the Internet chiefly as a source of background information and support.

- If infertility is causing you severe depression or anxiety, search out professional psychological counseling. Ask your doctor or call RESOLVE for a referral.
- If infertility is causing continuous severe problems between you and your partner, consider joint therapy with a trained counselor *who specializes in treating infertile couples.* Check with RESOLVE for referrals to mental health professionals who work regularly with infertile couples. If your partner won't join you, go alone.

Use Relaxation Skills to Cope with Infertility Treatment

Much of the rest of this book describes the medical technology available today for women and men with infertility. These treatments are now standard at infertility clinics everywhere in the United States. Most couples start with the simplest and least expensive approaches, such as the woman taking drugs like clomiphene or gonadotropins to stimulate ovulation. If these approaches do not succeed, you can choose to move up, one step at a time, to the more sophisticated assisted reproductive methods such as IVF, ICSI, GIFT, and ZIFT.

Many couples cope well with drug regimens, and good fertility clinics are organized to keep stress and discomfort to a relative minimum. And if you are lucky and become pregnant within a relatively short time, you may not become unusually stressed by the experience. However, if you end up continuing with treatments month after month and year after year, the depressing downside of the failures, the discomforts, and the psychological roller coaster of hopes up and hopes crashed not surprisingly can lead to chronic depression and anxiety.

JAN'S STORY

We put off having a baby for what we thought were responsible reasons. Knowing we deliberately did that has been difficult for me. And I'm wondering why we bothered, why we thought we had so much control over our fertility. I know now I don't have much control and neither do the doctors, despite what you hear and read.

It's been difficult for my husband, too, but everything seems centered on my body. He's a bit detached, but he's also disappointed. It's also hard for him to see someone he loves suffering and to know he can't do anything about it. The second miscarriage was hard on him—it was as if he failed an important test.

One of the hardest parts of infertility is that it gets worse instead of better with the passing of time. I had an ectopic pregnancy to start with and it may have damaged my right fallopian tube. Then I had a second pregnancy and lost it. Every month that passes and every pregnancy that doesn't happen and each something else that goes wrong mean you have less chance of having a baby.

When you have a loss and then can't get pregnant, every month you're reminded again. You're experiencing the loss all over again and at the same time you're concerned about what's next—it's a rough combination. And the treatment can be so difficult. When the nurse warned me about side effects, that I might experience moodiness, I thought she meant I'd feel irritable. I had no idea what it would be like. I was in a deep, dark depression from the day after the first pill until two days after the last pill. I think only someone who's gone through this can know what it might be like.

This is the time when the relaxation response and mini-relaxations can vastly improve your ability to cope with the stress of medical appointments and procedures. Practiced daily, the relaxation response will help you get through each day with greater calm and balance, and will reduce the tensions that quickly accumulate.

Mini-relaxations, as we mentioned, are a great way to calm yourself when you don't have time to evoke the relaxation response. They're particularly helpful for coping with the anxious events of high-tech treatments, such as the ultrasound examination of your ovaries or the insertion of an intravenous needle, the egg retrieval and transfer phase of IVF, and before you go into the bathroom on day 28 of your cycle to see if your period has started. They're especially useful while waiting for the phone to ring with the results of a pregnancy test.

In addition, you should remember that if you are taking hormonal drugs for your infertility you may experience rapid and unpredictable mood changes. If you notice that you're frequently upset with yourself and others, consider the infertility drugs you're taking. Question your doctor about side effects and don't hesitate to call if you're experiencing an effect that wasn't mentioned. Simply being aware of the fallout from these drugs will make you feel less out of control. You also can ask the people who are most likely to feel the brunt of your mood swings to bear with you while you're under treatment.

QUESTIONS TO ASK YOUR DOCTOR

❧ If I decide that I am having difficulty coping, is there a therapist you can recommend who is well versed in the emotional aspects of infertility?

❧ Is there a local infertility support group leader you recommend?

❧ Will you support me in using relaxation techniques during procedures, including bringing a portable tape player into a procedure or operating room?

❧ Do you have any patients whose medical situations are similar to mine whom I can talk to?

Step 5:
Take Advantage of Nature—
Tests and Medications That Help

If you've tried the suggestions we made in Steps 1 and 4, and still haven't been able to conceive, you may be wondering how long you should continue such strategies and when it would be appropriate to go to the next step. If you are in your late thirties or early forties, and the fact that you're not conceiving is weighing on your mind, or if there's a little voice in your head that wonders if everything possible is being done to help you get pregnant, it may be time to seek a specialist. We'd like to note that it's very useful for a couple to go to an infertility specialist. And for many, a fertility center is a good choice because it offers centralized, up-to-date care for both partners.

As you and your partner prepare to check out infertility treatments—or even before you do—we feel it's not too soon to begin thinking and talking about several issues: how far you want to go with treatments and, if they don't succeed, what do you see in your future? How do you feel about adoption? About egg or sperm donation? About having a child-free life? These are not decisions anyone can make overnight, which is why we raise them with our patients early in the process of trying to resolve their infertility.

If you choose to try treatment, you may find that what you have learned about the mind/body interaction will stand you in good stead as you proceed. Good nutrition and moderate exercise will continue to enhance your reproductive capabilities. And the techniques of relaxation, mindfulness, pleasing yourself, partner communication, and learning to say no that you acquire in a support group or mind/body intervention program will be invaluable aids during treatments. Many of the tapes listed in the Appendix (pages 231–234) are useful for helping to elicit the relaxation response and other relaxation techniques, especially when you're feeling stressed by a treatment or by its failure in that cycle. The Extended Relaxation Exercise/Beach Walk tape (page 232) is particularly good to listen to during medical or surgical procedures. And what you learn about tuning in to your body and mind can be a terrific support not only while you are trying to conceive, but afterward as well, when you're trying to keep up with an energetic child.

Finding a Specialist

If you haven't been able to get pregnant after several months or more of trying, where—and how soon—do you go for help? If you are a woman over the age of thirty-five, or have had a reproductive health problem such as a sexually transmitted disease, pelvic inflammatory disease, endometriosis, pelvic surgery, or very irregular menstrual cycles, it may be wise to seek expert help after only a few months of trying, rather than wait for twelve months to pass, which has been the conventional advice given younger women. (This is the advice given by RESOLVE, based on its extensive experience with infertile couples.) Many infertile women say they wish they'd been more aggressive in looking for expert assistance—and had done it sooner.

Although your first inclination may be to talk to your own gynecologist and urologist, the experience of many couples makes it clear that you need to be thoughtful about which source of expertise you select. It would be helpful to evaluate the clinical training and the focus of the practice of the physician you are considering for infertility services and advice. You can do this by drafting a list of questions and by actively making inquiries among as many resources as you can find, such as RESOLVE, the Internet, or other couples experiencing infertility. In addition, at the end of this chapter you'll find a list of questions that may help (see pages 148–149).

You can go to your obstetrician/gynecologist for infertility assistance or you can find a certified infertility specialist or fertility center. Obstetrician/gynecologists train for four years in primary care, gynecology, obstetrics, reproductive cancers, high-risk obstetrics, and infertility. In contrast, certified infertility specialists (more formally called reproductive endocrinologists) have trained for six or seven years, with at least two or three years of that time focused in infertility treatment. The extra training provides the time they need to acquire the necessary specialized medical skills.

An up-to-date list of certified infertility specialists is available at the Web site of the American Society for Reproductive Medicine/Society of Reproductive Endocrinologists at www.socrei.org. Infertility specialists are listed by state and city. Most of these specialists focus on treating infertile couples; some ob/gyns are similarly focused: their extensive experience enables them to provide care that's comparable to a certified infertility specialist.

At the same time it's a good idea for the male partner to be checked by a urologist who specializes in infertility problems or by an andrologist, who specializes in male reproductive disorders related to the hormonal system. This is especially important if the partner has had a sexually transmitted disease.

The best sources for referrals for infertility diagnosis and treatment are medical schools, large group medical practices, health maintenance organizations, large hospitals, and RESOLVE. RESOLVE has available the names of almost eight hundred physicians in the United States and Canada who are fully trained and certified in reproductive endocrinology and whose education and credentials fulfill criteria developed by RESOLVE. Their performance is regularly reviewed by an independent board. The list also includes urologists who have had extra training in treating male infertility and who meet RESOLVE criteria.

The entire list of physicians is available to RESOLVE members; nonmembers who telephone its helpline at 617-623-0744 will be given the names of two doctors in a specific locality. If you want to check independently on whether a physician is board certified in a particular specialty, you can call the American Board of Medical Specialties at 800-776-2378, or try the Internet at www.certifieddoctor.org, and select the "verification" option that's offered. It's usually not wise to choose an infertility specialist from the telephone book without learning more about him or her.

ELIZABETH'S STORY

I went to my own gynecologist when I had trouble getting pregnant after a miscarriage. He had my FSH levels tested, but on day 5, not on day 3. When he saw the results he told me I was going into menopause. I was shocked—I was only thirty-four years old. He wanted me to quickly go on ovulation-stimulating drugs. I didn't know what to do. I was already so distraught after my miscarriage that I was just numb. It was my husband who insisted we get a second opinion and go to an infertility center. When I was tested at the center my hormone levels were found to be normal. My husband was tested for the first time and his tests also were normal.

I have what is called unexplained infertility. I feel sad, hopeless,

and exhausted all the time. If I only knew why I can't get pregnant
I think I could get on with my life. I didn't realize until it hap-
pened that my self-esteem is tied to my ability to conceive. I have
such a sense of failure, of having no value.

I wish I'd chosen to see an infertility specialist much sooner
than I did and had been more of an advocate for myself. I'd
strongly recommend that other infertile women take time to think
through their medical decisions despite their desire to become
pregnant as soon as possible.

Because infertility can have a variety of complex causes and can
affect either partner, fertility centers, with their teams of specialists, generally are considered better able to provide the skills and
resources necessary not only for assisted reproduction but also for
all the stages of infertility treatment, including a thorough diagnostic workup of both partners.

At first, the quality of fertility clinics was highly variable, and
when quoting their rates of IVF success, they did not differentiate
between live births and conceptions. Now all are using live births
as their measure of success. Because the number of such centers in
the United States was growing so rapidly ten years ago, it appeared
necessary that they be licensed. Today they are under the purview
of the U.S. Centers for Disease Control (CDC). Unannounced site
visits are made to check the quality of their operations and the
validity of their success rates. The CDC publishes the results of
these surveys, making it possible for you to read a one-page summary report on any fertility center you're considering. Almost all
centers are represented. The CDC report *Assisted Reproductive*
Technology Success Rates: National Summary and Fertility Clinic
Reports is available from the Division of Reproductive Health,
Centers for Disease Control, 4770 Buford Highway, Atlanta, GA
30341-3714. It also can be found on the RESOLVE Web page at

www.resolve.org. Simply highlight the name of the report.

Today, by using the information gathered by the CDC, plus the useful "Questions to Ask" fact sheet published by RESOLVE, you can make your search for a quality clinic more focused and less time consuming. This approach improves your chances of finding a high-quality physician and/or clinic. If you get the CDC report, pay particular attention to its introduction and the section "Other Factors to Consider." In addition, bear in mind that clinics' performance levels can change quickly and published data usually is two or more years old.

We would like to note that no matter how reputable the clinic or doctor, it is always a good idea for couples to get a second opinion after a diagnosis or upon completion of infertility tests. Simply request copies of your record and X rays (it is usually not necessary to repeat tests) for the purpose of consultation.

CAUSES OF INFERTILITY

A recent review of the cases of 14,000 couples demonstrated that the causes of infertility can be broken down roughly into fourths: a little over one-fourth are due to ovulation disorders or a depleted supply of eggs; another fourth are due to low sperm counts; a little less than one-fourth are the result of tubal dysfunction or blockage; and the last fourth are from other causes such as endometriosis, uterine fibroids, genetics, or problems that can't be explained.

Causes of Infertility

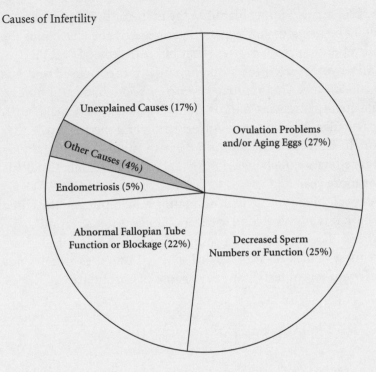

Because ovulation disorders and sperm abnormalities are such common causes of infertility, the first tests you have (or will do yourself) will be those described in Step 3, basic evaluations to determine whether you and your partner are producing eggs and sperm. If sperm tests are normal, and basal body temperature and an LH surge test indicate that ovulation does occur, you will probably be told to go home and have intercourse regularly, such as every other day, for the three to five days before and up to the estimated day of ovulation. If this approach doesn't succeed after a few months, it may be time for a more detailed workup for both of you. How soon you pursue the further identification of infertility factors is a personal decision. *In general, the older the woman is,*

the faster a couple should move to the next steps of infertility diagnosis and treatment.

Tests for Ovulation

There are four relatively simple methods for discovering whether you are ovulating. A menstrual cycle that's shorter than twenty-two days or longer than thirty-five days can be an indication of a mild ovulatory problem. And you can chart your own basal body temperature and/or test your urine with a drugstore LH monitoring kit, to learn for yourself whether or not you are ovulating. See Step 3, pages 61–66, for a description.

The fourth method, a blood test, can be performed to determine whether your progesterone becomes elevated seven to ten days after the LH surge that triggers ovulation. A blood analysis showing an elevated progesterone level suggests that a normal ovulation probably occurred.

It's possible to use ultrasound to determine whether ovulation appears to have taken place, and to perform an endometrial biopsy to make certain the lining of your uterus is ready at just the right time to accept a fertilized egg. However, these are expensive and, in the case of a biopsy, carry a slight risk of complications. They are used chiefly to help pin down a puzzling cause for a lack of ovulation. They are not necessary if the other four tests demonstrate that ovulation is taking place.

The ultrasound used today at fertility centers visualizes the ovaries and/or uterus from inside the abdomen via a slim, gel-coated probe that's inserted into the vagina. Ultrasound is a safe diagnostic tool because its images are produced by sound waves, not radiation.

REASONS FOR IMPAIRED OVULATION

If these tests find that you aren't ovulating, the reason is likely to be due to fluctuations in the hypothalamus/pituitary system that governs your ovaries. As we noted in Step 2, the tiny hypothalamus area of your brain directs the function of both the nervous and the hormonal systems of your body. It can be influenced by emotional events and other life experiences, including diet, stress, and depression. The hypothalamus converts signals from your nerves into hormonal signals. It communicates with the nearby pituitary gland through the nerves and the short stalk of blood vessels that connect these two glands and carry hormones from one to the other. It also is affected by levels of the hormones produced by the ovaries and other parts of the reproductive system.

During your monthly menstrual cycle the complex process of ovulation begins when the hypothalamus secretes a hormone called gonadotropin-releasing hormone (GnRH) that goes to the pituitary. The GnRH signals the pituitary to start producing and releasing follicle-stimulating hormone (FSH) and luteinizing hormone (LH). (These two hormones are called gonadotropins because they affect the gonads—ovaries in women and testes in men.) Regular pulses of large amounts of FSH—a pulse about every sixty to ninety minutes—stimulate follicle growth in the female and sperm production in the male.

As the ovaries receive FSH, some follicles will respond and grow larger but, generally, after two or three days, one follicle becomes dominant—it grows larger than the others and the egg it contains begins to mature. This follicle also is responsible for secreting most of the estrogen that circulates in your blood during this follicular phase—the first half—of your monthly cycle. The dominant follicle reaches its maximum size—about one inch in diameter—just before ovulation (in a twenty-eight-day cycle, this would be about day 12). At this point, the estrogen it has secreted triggers the pituitary to pulse out a surge of LH, which signals the follicle to ovulate, to slowly open up and release the egg one or two days later.

After ovulation, the empty follicle forms a type of cyst called the corpus luteum, which secretes progesterone as well as estrogen. The progesterone affects the uterus, causing it to prepare for the possibility of a pregnancy. This is called the luteal phase of your cycle.

The Hypothalamus/Pituitary System

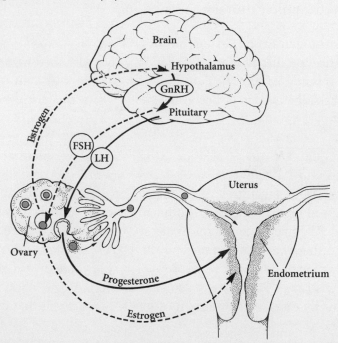

The hypothalamus area of the brain directs the hormonal system. It is influenced by many external events including emotions, stress, and diet, as well as hormones from other parts of the reproductive system. The hypothalamus secretes gonadotropin-releasing hormone (GnRH), which signals the nearby pituitary gland to produce follicle-stimulating hormone (FSH) and luteinizing hormone (LH). These enter the bloodstream and, when they reach the ovaries, stimulate the growth of an egg cell and ovulation. After ovulation, the ovaries produce higher levels of progesterone and estradiol, which promote endometrial growth in the uterus and reset the hypothalamus/pituitary cycle.

Not surprisingly, this finely tuned, hormonally driven interaction among the hypothalamus, the pituitary, and the ovaries is the most frequent source of problems in women who aren't ovulating regularly. The delicate balance of this system may not function correctly due to a number of causes or, in rarer instances, it may never have gotten under way at all.

Hypothalamic/Pituitary Dysfunction

A dysfunction of this system not only is the most common of all ovulation problems, it also is the most easily corrected with infertility therapy. After treatment for this problem a woman usually has the same chance of becoming pregnant as any fertile woman of her age.

The relationship between the hypothalamus, pituitary, and ovaries can get out of balance fairly easily. As we mentioned in Steps 1 and 4, if you weigh too much or too little, if you don't have enough body fat, if you're exercising too rigorously, or if you're depressed or stressed, the hypothalamus and pituitary may be affected. The hypothalamic/pituitary system is designed to be sensitive to these various stimuli and the usual cascade of hormonal events may be altered in response. As a result, you may not ovulate or menstruate. This system also can be affected by genetic disorders or by disease, including tumors, if they disturb that area of the brain.

ARE YOU TAKING A PSYCHOACTIVE DRUG?

Drugs such as antidepressants and other psychoactive medications can change the normal levels of various hormones and interfere with ovulation. It's important to discuss these possible effects with your physician, although today most medical experts believe that if you are clinically depressed, it is better to stay on an antidepressant than put yourself at risk of a relapse.

Polycystic Ovarian Syndrome

Perhaps the most frequent cause of hypothalamic/pituitary dysfunction is polycystic ovarian syndrome, or PCOS. It's termed polycystic because it characteristically produces an excess of small follicles (smaller than a pea) in the ovaries. In PCOS, many follicles start to develop, but none becomes fully developed and ovulation doesn't occur. Women with PCOS usually have had years of irregular menstrual cycles, starting in their teens, often fewer than six cycles a year. They may also have acne and excessive hair on their faces or chests. The elevated levels of LH, testosterone, and insulin that this disorder causes can be measured in the blood and used as clues to determine how to correct such imbalances so that the ovaries will respond appropriately.

Less Common Ovulation Problems

It's possible for a woman to ovulate regularly yet never become pregnant because her uterus doesn't have enough time to get ready to nurture an embryo. *Luteal phase defect,* as it's called, occurs when the endometrium develops four or more days too late to be acceptable to an embryo. A "mature" endometrium is thick with the blood vessels needed to supply an embryo nourishment as it undergoes its rapid development. If necessary, the maturity of the uterine lining can be determined by taking a biopsy of its tissue.

As a dominant follicle enlarges, it normally produces steadily increasing amounts of estrogen that stimulate the endometrium to grow. An ultrasound made at the time of ovulation usually reveals an endometrium that already has become 8 to 12 mm thick, if it's developing normally. If this growth is delayed, the cause may be insufficient stimulation before ovulation. Or, after ovulation, the corpus luteum doesn't secrete enough progesterone for endometrial development. The causes of luteal phase defect usually can be treated successfully with drugs.

In rare instances, an endometrial biopsy may be needed to determine whether the lining of the uterus is sufficiently developed in time to nurture the fertilized egg when it's likely to arrive, about six days after ovulation. To perform such a biopsy, done in the doctor's office, a tiny sample of tissue is suctioned from the lining, using a catheter that creates a small amount of suction. This procedure usually causes a sharp cramp. There may be mild cramps afterward and some spotting for a few days.

Premature Ovarian Failure

Another reason for lack of ovulation may be ovaries that aren't working because they don't have enough follicles and eggs or because the follicles have aged prematurely and no longer respond to follicle-stimulating hormone (FSH). An unchangeable aspect of the ovaries is that the number of follicles and eggs they contain is fixed before birth and then almost immediately begins to decrease. At the time of birth most human ovaries hold approximately one million eggs. By the time a woman starts ovulating, that number has dropped to about 250,000 and continues to decrease markedly. Only 300 to 500 eggs actually mature and are ovulated during a woman's reproductive life. Usually one oocyte matures each month in a follicle on the ovary's surface; it appears that the follicles most sensitive to FSH are the first to respond to its stimulation.

As a woman and her ovaries grow older, apparently what remains in the ovaries are the follicles that have been somewhat resistant to the promptings of FSH. And the eggs in these aging follicles are less likely to result in a successful pregnancy. The chief reason is that the machinery of those aging cells is not working properly. Their chromosomes may be damaged and the nutrients in the cell may be exhausted. Researchers feel it's possible that the time-associated decrease in a woman's ability to become pregnant is due to a decline in both the quantity and quality of her eggs, as well as their lack of responsiveness to FSH.

Diagnosing Ovarian Failure: Day 3 FSH

As we said, the pituitary begins to release pulses of LH and FSH as you begin to menstruate, on the first day of your menstrual cycle. Usually one follicle responds to this stimulation, and when large enough, it secretes sufficient estradiol estrogen to turn down the FSH pulses. As time passes, however, the follicles that remain in the ovaries are likely to be those not very sensitive to FSH, so more and more of that hormone is secreted by the pituitary in an effort to goad a follicle into action. If no follicle enlarges, the pituitary keeps on pumping out FSH, raising the blood levels of this hormone with each day of the menstrual cycle. The amount of FSH in blood drawn on day 3 of the cycle is an indicator of whether FSH levels are normal or high. (FSH levels peak on day 2, 3, or 4; day 3 has been chosen chiefly because it's the middle day.)

A recent study of in vitro fertilization results showed an ongoing pregnancy rate of 18 percent among women who had normal levels of FSH on the third day of their cycles. In contrast, women with an abnormally high day 3 FSH had a pregnancy rate of zero. Some reproductive endocrinologists believe that day 3 FSH and a woman's age are important predictors of a woman's ability to get pregnant.

If you are over thirty-five and haven't conceived after six months of trying, many fertility specialists recommend that you have a day 3 FSH blood test. Some even believe that this test should be done for infertile women as young as thirty.

Clomiphene Challenge Test

Another, even more informative assessment of the responsiveness of the ovaries is the clomiphene citrate challenge test. After a day 3 FSH test, the woman takes a 100 mg clomiphene tablet on days 5 through 9, a blood sample is drawn on day 10, and the test for FSH is repeated. If either of the two blood tests shows an elevated level, it can be assumed that her supply of eggs is depleted. Some fertility centers find that the clomiphene challenge test is more informative than the day 3 test alone, since as many as 75 percent of women whose egg supply is somewhat reduced will have normal day 3 FSH levels.

Women with fewer, less responsive follicles need to start fertility treatments sooner rather than later. If their egg/follicle supply is exhausted, they still may be able to become pregnant with the help of a donor egg fertilized by their partner's sperm.

Genetic, lifestyle, and environmental factors all may play a role in determining the rate at which your follicle pool diminishes. Cigarette smoking, for example, appears to hasten the pace at which the number of follicles is depleted, and menopause occurs measurably earlier in women who smoke.

Congenital Conditions

Congenital conditions also can prevent normal reproduction. Most commonly seen is *Turner's syndrome*, which affects approximately one in three thousand baby girls. The child is born with forty-five instead of forty-six chromosomes, and the missing one is the X chromosome needed for female sexual characteristics. These girls tend to be short, have differences in their eyes and bones, and have narrowed aortas. At puberty, these girls may not develop breasts or other secondary sexual characteristics and may not menstruate.

Another inborn condition is *ovarian dysgenesis,* or the lack of eggs and ovaries. Women who have this disorder have a uterus but no ovaries. Although they aren't able to have a child who carries their biological component, they can become pregnant with a fertilized donor egg and give birth.

Other Tests

Many physicians prefer to make certain that fallopian tubes are open and semen and sperm are normal before starting their patients on a drug regimen. Fallopian tubes are examined with an X-ray test called hysterosalpingogram (HSG) in which a dye visible by X ray is injected into the uterus to reveal its shape and whether the tubes are unobstructed. HSG is described in detail in Step 6A, pages 153–154. Sperm health also should be evaluated before a course of treatment is discussed.

TREATMENTS

It is worth mentioning again that before treatment is undertaken, it is a good idea to take a copy of your test results to another doctor or clinic for a second opinion.

We feel that the evaluations and treatments for infertility should be done one step at a time, with the less invasive (and least expensive) performed first and the invasive and more specialized procedures resorted to only after conservative treatment has not succeeded. Furthermore, couples should take three to six months after each therapy to allow pregnancy to occur.

THE STAIRCASE APPROACH TO TREATMENT

Step 1. Identify all factors that might be contributing to infertility.
Step 2. Correct all the factors that are found.
Step 3. Try either clomiphene citrate or intrauterine insemination (IUI) alone; if not successful, use clomiphene and IUI together. (IUI is described in Step 6A, pages 161–164.)
Step 4. Move to human menopausal gonadotropin, often combined with IUI.
Step 5. Move to assisted reproductive technologies.

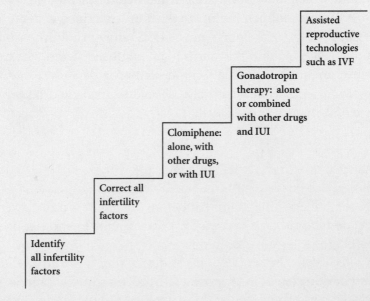

Women who have a healthy reproductive tract but are not ovulating because of hormonal reasons have the greatest success with infertility therapy. The treatments chosen, of course, depend largely on the source of the problem. Nondrug methods include weight gain or loss regimens, stress reduction programs, efforts to treat preexisting depression, and cessation or severe modification of an exercise regimen. Drug treatments to restore ovulation include the use of clomiphene citrate pills alone or combined with intrauterine insemination, clomiphene citrate plus other hormone drugs, or gonadotropin injections. If a woman's prolactin levels are higher than normal, bromocriptine is indicated. Each of these drugs may be combined with intrauterine insemination.

The chance of conceiving, however, also may depend on other factors, such as age, the quality of the partner's sperm, the normalcy of the cervical mucus, and the woman's overall health. After age thirty-five a woman's response to infertility drugs may become reduced; at age forty it may drop even more sharply.

If the less invasive steps in treatment are not successful, many couples choose to stop at this point and consider other options such as adopting or building a life that does not include children. Others, however, may wish to go further before choosing these alternatives. They might explore assisted reproductive technologies such as in vitro fertilization (IVF), in which the egg is fertilized in the laboratory and the developing embryo is placed in the mother's uterus, or gamete intrafallopian transfer (GIFT), in which the egg and sperm are inserted into the fallopian tube, or the several variations of these methods. Such technologies are covered in the chapter "Extra Steps."

Clomiphene Citrate

Clomiphene citrate (brand names: Clomid, Serophene) primarily affects the hypothalamus, causing an increase in the body's pulses of gonadotropin-releasing hormone, which in turn causes increased FSH and LH secretion. For clomiphene citrate to be effective, you need to be already producing a somewhat normal level of estrogen, your ovaries must be able to function, and your hypothalamus and pituitary must be able to secrete their hormones. If you aren't menstruating, it'll be necessary to induce menstruation. Clomiphene is most effective in women who have a hypothalamic/pituitary dysfunction, which we described on page 132.

Clomiphene is usually given in a 50 mg pill and taken every day for five continuous days per cycle. It is started on cycle day 3, 4, or 5 after menstruation. About 50 percent of women who are good candidates for this treatment will ovulate at the 50 mg per day dose. Another 25 percent will ovulate if the dose is increased to 100 mg a day. This drug generally is used for no more than three to six cycles; after the third cycle clomiphene citrate treatment begins to become less effective. If you try clomiphene and don't become pregnant after six cycles, your physician should look for other possible causes of infertility and discuss alternative drug treatments with you.

In most instances, ovulation occurs five to twelve days after the last dose of clomiphene. To increase their chances of conceiving, couples can have intercourse frequently (every other day, for example) after cycle day 10, or may use an ovulation test kit to pinpoint more exactly the best time to have sex. Blood tests or ultrasound are available for those who want greater certainty about ovulation.

Although the Food and Drug Administration has approved the use of clomiphene citrate up to 100 mg daily, in certain instances many reproductive endocrinologists have been using the drug safely at doses of 150 mg, 200 mg, or even up to 250 mg per day. Women who fail to ovulate at the lower doses may ovulate at these higher ones; in fact, up to 70 percent of those who don't ovulate at lower doses will ovulate at the higher dose, but fewer than 30 percent become pregnant.

Side Effects

Some side effects have been reported by women treated with clomiphene citrate. The rate of miscarriage after a clomiphene-induced pregnancy appears to be 15 to 25 percent, which is similar to the rates reported by all infertile couples, regardless of treatment. The incidence of birth defects is no different from that of fertile couples. More common side effects include hot flushes in about 20 percent of women and enlarged ovaries in about 15 percent. A smaller percentage of women will experience abdominal discomfort, often caused by their swollen ovaries. Other side effects that may not be serious but still can make life distinctly uncomfortable are mood swings that can be extreme, breast tenderness, headaches, nervousness, dizziness, nausea and vomiting, and fatigue. A woman who experiences visual disturbances such as blurry vision or a blind spot should stop taking the clomiphene and contact her doctor.

In addition, there's a slight risk with clomiphene therapy of having multiple babies. About 8 percent of women who take clomiphene citrate have twins and just under one percent have triplets. Because clomiphene is used so frequently, however, the number of triplet births that result has been substantial.

Clomiphene Citrate Plus

If a series of clomiphene treatments alone doesn't induce ovulation, this drug can be combined with others to enhance its effectiveness. One of the most common additions is a single injection of human chorionic gonadotropin (hCG). In some instances we check follicle development with ultrasound and give the injection when the follicle reaches more than 20 mm (about one inch) in size. Clomiphene citrate also can be combined with glucosteroids such as prednisone to increase the rate of ovulation and pregnancy successfully in women who have elevated levels of the adrenal androgen DHEAS and fail to ovulate with standard clomiphene treatment.

For those women who respond poorly to either clomiphene or gonadotropin therapy, a combination of these two drugs sometimes proves effective in triggering ovulation.

Human Menopausal Gonadotropin (hMG)

As we mentioned in Step 2, gonadotropins stimulate the gonads, which in women mean the ovaries. Next to clomiphene citrate, human menopausal gonadotropins are another step in encouraging follicles to develop when a woman's own hormone system is not doing the job. Two brands (Humegon and Repronex) are derived from the urine of postmenopausal women, which is distilled into highly purified preparations containing both FSH and LH. Someone other than the recipient administers a daily injection into the muscles of the buttocks or hip. Repronex also can be injected under the skin. This therapy is much more expensive than clomiphene treatment—each cycle typically costs $800 to $2000, compared to $50 to $100 for a clomiphene cycle.

Treatment is started usually two or three days after the beginning of menstruation and continued until cycle day 7. At this point a blood test is made to measure the level of estradiol estrogen. If the level is not high enough, the dose of gonadotropin usually must be increased to meet that woman's need. If there's too much response to the drug, the dose should be reduced until the appropriate serum estradiol level is reached to avoid follicle overstimulation. In addition, ultrasound is used to follow follicle development. When estradiol levels are in the correct range and one or two follicles are sufficiently developed, human chorionic gonadotropin (hCG) is injected as a substitute for LH to trigger ovulation. It is so similar to LH that it can be used as a replacement for it. Ovulation usually occurs within thirty-six hours. If estradiol levels are very high and/or four or more follicles develop, hCG usually is not given and the cycle is cancelled in order to avoid the risk of multiple fetuses or ovarian overstimulation.

Other gonadotropin preparations that are being used today (Follistim and Gonal-F) are manufactured by laboratories using recombinant DNA technology. They're injected under the skin, like a diabetic's insulin shot.

Many clinical studies have evaluated gonadotropin therapies and most found few important differences in effectiveness and safety among the treatments. A woman who receives this treatment has about a 90 percent chance of ovulating and, if she does ovulate, about a 25 percent chance of becoming pregnant during each cycle, which is the pregnancy rate of a fertile woman. Again, age is a factor in the pregnancy rate. After three cycles of treatment most women who are able to become pregnant by this method will have conceived. Except for women who have polycystic ovarian syndrome (PCOS), the choice of therapy usually depends on the physician's experience with the drugs or on the patient's preference regarding cost and the route of injection. For women with PCOS, however, a low-dose, long-term FSH-only gonadotropin therapy is better than high-dose FSH treatment because it reduces the risk of excessive ovarian stimulation.

Side Effects

This therapy produces some mild side effects such as irritation at the site of the injection, requiring the use of different sites. Cervical mucus might become heavy, and fatigue, mood swings, headaches, bloating, abdominal pain, and weight gain can make life uncomfortable for women receiving gonadotropin therapy.

There also are major risks of gonadotropin therapy: an increased chance of having a multiple-embryo pregnancy and of experiencing mild or even severe ovarian hyperstimulation. The multiple pregnancy rate is approximately 20 percent, with twins being most common. The chance of developing more than two or three embryos is reduced by administering low doses over a two- to three-week period.

The development of many embryos often results when women are not content with such an approach and choose to hurry the therapy and take the chance of having a high multiple pregnancy. When this occurs, there is a substantial risk of losing some or all of the babies because there isn't enough room in the womb for them to develop. Those who survive may be premature and face the problems most preemies have. To help ensure that at least some of the babies will survive, many women with multiple embryos choose to have the number of fetuses decreased through selective reduction.

Mild ovarian enlargement, sometimes accompanied by abdominal symptoms, is experienced by roughly 20 percent of women receiving gonadotropin therapy. Severe ovarian hyperstimulation is rare, occurring in about 1.3 percent of patients. Symptoms of both the severe and mild forms of ovarian stimulation typically begin to develop five to seven days after ovulation is triggered. These may include abdominal pain and distention, nausea, vomiting, diarrhea, and difficulty in breathing. Women receiving this therapy should be carefully monitored with frequent blood tests and ultrasound so that the drug dose can be adjusted to prevent side effects. Regardless of what the tests show, however, women should be alert to the first sign of ovarian/abdominal distress and report it right away to their physicians.

Unless there are serious complications, bed rest and pain medication are the most useful interventions for easing symptoms of ovarian hyperstimulation. Most cases subside in one to two weeks.

Bromocriptine

This drug (brand name: Parlodel) is the treatment of choice for infertile women who do not ovulate, ovulate very infrequently, or have luteal phase defect, and whose blood tests reveal that their pituitary glands are secreting excessive amounts of prolactin. The pituitary ordinarily releases high levels of prolactin during pregnancy and after the birth of a baby to stimulate the breasts to make milk. It also interferes with normal ovulation or the normal luteal phase, which is why women who are nursing exclusively often don't ovulate.

A high level of prolactin in women who are not pregnant can have many causes, such as antidepressants, blood pressure pills, an anesthetic, stress, excessive exercise, or an underactive thyroid. Most frequently, however, the cause is a benign growth in the pituitary gland.

Bromocriptine is a form of ergotamine that suppresses prolactin production. Because it can produce side effects easily, it is started with a very low dose (one-quarter of a tablet), given once a day at bedtime at first, and then increased gradually. Blood should be tested again for prolactin levels after four to eight weeks of treatment. The lowest dose possible needed to keep prolactin levels normal should be used. After prolactin secretion becomes normal, if ovulation doesn't resume after approximately two months of this therapy, an additional boost from either clomiphene or gonadotropin therapy may be included. If conception doesn't take place after four to six months of ovulation, it's time to rethink the process and perhaps start the steps of treatment again from the beginning. For women who are suitable candidates for bromocriptine therapy, the pregnancy rate is about 80 percent.

Side Effects

If started in the way we just described, most women do very well on bromocriptine, but some may experience side effects. The most common generally are unpleasant but not serious: light-headedness, nausea, diarrhea, vomiting, fatigue, the feeling of being unwell, headache, runny nose, and watery eyes. If these become too distressing, it may be worth taking the drug by placing the pill in the vagina. Some studies—not all—have seen fewer side effects with this approach.

Fertility Drugs and the Risks of Ovarian Cancer

Ovulation-inducing drugs have been in use since the late 1950s. Over four hundred studies have looked at their adverse reactions and long- and short-term side effects, including cancer. Only two studies, in 1992 and 1994, found any effects that could be considered health threatening to either the women taking these drugs or to the children born after their use. These two studies found an increased risk of ovarian tumors among women who had been given fertility drugs.

The 1992 research found that an infertile woman who took such drugs and did not have a baby had a greater chance of developing ovarian cancer than did a woman who hadn't taken the drugs. We should add, however, that questions have been raised about the design of this study.

The second research project reviewed the medical histories of 3800 women who had used clomiphene and found eleven cases of ovarian tumors among them. Of the eleven tumors, seven were benign or borderline tumors of the ovary and four actually were cancers. Borderline here means the growths were neither clearly benign nor clearly malignant. The incidence of four cancers was similar to the number of cancers expected in an average population of women—about one per 1000 women. Ovarian tumors can be found by ultrasound.

The incidence of borderline tumors, however, was higher than normal. A review of the data showed that the women who had developed borderline tumors had taken clomiphene for at least twelve consecutive cycles. As a result, fertility specialists generally avoid using clomiphene for so many cycles.

Our current view of this data is that infertility or childlessness (voluntary or involuntary) is a more important risk factor for ovarian tumors than treatment with an ovulation-inducing medication. *Nevertheless, you as a patient should be aware that if clomiphene citrate isn't effective after six cycles, your physician should consider other methods of inducing ovulation, such as gonadotropins.*

Surgical Treatment of PCOS

Women who have polycystic ovarian syndrome that has not responded to weight loss or clomiphene citrate treatment have several choices for the next stage of therapy: in vitro fertilization, gonadotropin drugs (and the possibility of multiple fetuses), or surgery to rectify the condition. Before the advent of fertility drugs, surgically removing wedges of ovarian tissue was a common method of restoring ovulation. Because it often led to adhesions between the ovary and fallopian tube, this operation fell into disfavor. Today, however, it's been replaced with a technique that uses laparoscopy and a laser beam or electrocautery to puncture the surface of the ovary in a number of places, destroying much of the ovarian tissue that makes testosterone. The operation is done as an outpatient laparoscopy, takes about thirty-five minutes or so, and requires a day or two of recovery. It also requires general anesthesia, however, and costs about $5000. It may be covered by some insurance plans.

Destroying the tissue inhibits the ovary's overproduction of male hormones for approximately eight to twelve months, allowing ovulation to occur during that time. After such surgery, the twelve-month pregnancy rate is found to be 50 to 60 percent. When the ovarian tissue grows back, however, PCOS recurs. Long-term complications are few but do include the chance that scar tissue and adhesions might develop. This surgical treatment may be chosen by women who don't like the side effects of fertility drugs and are not interested in IVF.

If Your Problem Is Anatomical

Because anatomical irregularities of the reproductive tract also are a common cause of infertility, your physician will check its health during your basic diagnostic workup. Flaws in this part of your anatomy that were caused by inborn abnormalities, previous surgery, or disease often can be corrected—or bypassed—to lead to pregnancy. These problems and the methods available for correcting them are described in the next chapter.

QUESTIONS TO ASK YOUR DOCTOR

✧ Do you specialize in infertility diagnosis and treatment?

✧ Have you completed a fellowship in such diagnosis and treatment?

✧ Do you have a subspecialty certification in reproductive endocrinology and infertility?

- At what age does a woman's fertility begin to decline? A man's?

- What are the most important tests for both of us?

- Are they painful?

- What do they cost? Are they covered by insurance?

- I'm already beginning to feel anxious and depressed about not being able to have a baby. What can I do to manage these feelings better?

- If our tests don't show anything wrong, what do we do then?

- If I have an ovulation problem, how do you usually go about treating it?

- How many cycles do you usually recommend for each drug treatment?

- If a treatment isn't successful, what's next?

- What side effects are associated with these drugs?

Step 6A:
Find and Treat Anatomical Problems in the Woman

The health and normalcy of a woman's reproductive tract—her cervix, uterus, and fallopian tubes—are vital to her fertility. An unobstructed route through the cervix, uterus, and at least one tube is essential if sperm are to reach an egg after it's been gathered up by the nearest fallopian tube. Furthermore, each of these organs needs to be healthy and capable of carrying out its particular function if fertilization and pregnancy are to be successful.

The cervix is the gateway to your reproductive tract. The mucus it produces at the time of ovulation is essential because it shelters sperm from the acidity of the vagina. It also helps sperm enter the uterus and offers a protected environment for those that don't immediately move on.

A uterus that is abnormally shaped or has fibroids or scar tissue may not be able to provide the hospitable environment necessary to sustain an embryo. If its lining, the endometrium, doesn't develop fully or isn't ready at the time it's needed for the embryo (a problem called the luteal phase defect, discussed on pages 133–134), pregnancy can't take place.

A fallopian tube not only needs to be open, but it also must be lined with enough hairlike cilia to move the fertilized egg toward the uterus. It also must be lined with enough secretory cells to produce the protein-rich fluid that nurtures sperm, egg, and embryo while they're in the tube. It needs to be able to move its open end toward the ovary, and its fimbria should be sufficiently intact and mobile to help collect the egg from the surface of the ovary.

WHEN TUBES AREN'T OPEN

Fallopian tube problems are a fairly common reason for infertility. Almost all fallopian tube abnormalities occur during a woman's reproductive years and are the result of infection or pelvic surgery. Very few are congenital. In some instances, it's possible to correct a tubal problem surgically or with catheterization; in many others, however, surgery may not be successful.

The interior of each tube is extremely tiny, particularly the portion closest to the uterus, which has a diameter the size of a thread, just large enough for an embryo to slip through. Because this anatomy is so minute, the slightest amount of inflammation or ragged tissue can block an embryo's passage. The most common cause of tubal scarring and inflammation is pelvic inflammatory disease (PID), caused by one or more bouts of sexually transmitted diseases (STDs), chiefly chlamydia. Other inflammations, a ruptured appendix, an infection following an abortion, or previous tubal surgery occasionally may also lead to tubal scarring.

Pelvic Infections

A major cause of tubal problems, pelvic inflammatory disease occurs when a sexually transmitted disease spreads from the vagina into the upper reproductive tract, particularly to the fallopian tubes. Unfortunately, STDs—chlamydia, herpes simplex, gonorrhea, genital warts—are common among those who are sexually active; for example, about 3 million women and men become infected with chlamydia every year. A pelvic infection can develop after a single act of intercourse with a person who already has an STD. The chance of tubal infertility increases with each incidence of PID: after one episode the rate has been found to be 12 percent, after two episodes 23 percent, and after three the rate reaches 54 percent. It's possible to become infected over and over again and not be aware of it, especially with chlamydia. Many times the diseases that cause PID have no symptoms, or produce symptoms that occur late or aren't recognized. Chlamydia, for instance, is commonly a silent, symptomless STD, and many women and men don't know they're carrying it. It's often detected in the tissues of women who have tubal infertility.

Ruptured Appendix

Having had an appendix rupture sometime in the past can heighten a woman's chance of having a damaged tube. In one case-controlled study, a history of ruptured appendix was associated with a 4.8-fold increase in the risk of tubal infertility. Because it's so close by, an appendix inflammation can spread easily to the fallopian tubes and lead to scar tissue. Having appendicitis without rupture did not increase this risk.

Adhesions

Adhesions, which are permanent bridges of fibrous tissue, are created during what is otherwise a normal healing process. In the pelvic area, adhesions can cover the ovaries or the ends of the fallopian tubes, or can tightly connect the tubes to other structures so they can't move normally. Adhesions are found in approximately 75 percent of women who have had pelvic surgery.

Septic Abortion

It's possible for infection to develop after a miscarriage or the termination of a pregnancy, although it's uncommon, occurring in fewer than one percent of the cases. The resulting inflammation may leave scar tissue in the fallopian tubes that blocks or damages the interior of the tubes.

EXAMINING FALLOPIAN TUBES

The two most frequently used methods of examining the condition of your fallopian tubes are hysterosalpingography and laparoscopy.

Hysterosalpingography (HSG)

HSG is a basic test that's very accurate in most situations. It's usually performed between cycle days 6 and 11, before ovulation, to avoid the possibility of disrupting the movement of a fertilized egg through a tube or the uterus. While you are lying on your back under the X-ray machine, a catheter is threaded through your cervix into your uterus and a sterile contrast medium, a colorless "dye," is injected slowly through it. As the dye fills the uterus, X rays are taken every few seconds, revealing any abnormalities inside the uterus such as a divided cavity, fibroids, or adhesions. As dye begins to fill the fallopian tubes, more X rays are taken. If the tubes are open, eventually the dye leaks out the far end. If it stops anywhere in the tube, a blockage is indicated.

We should note that a certain number of HSGs are not always correct when they indicate a tubal blockage (a so-called false positive result), so a blockage usually should be confirmed by laparoscopy before any repair is undertaken. Such a false positive HSG often occurs when the uterine wall spasms in reaction to the contrast medium or the catheter. The spasm can close the fallopian tube where it joins the uterus, giving the impression there's a blockage at that juncture. Furthermore, an HSG doesn't provide information about the presence of problems *outside* the uterus, such as ovarian adhesions or endometriosis.

Many medical centers will prepare women before this procedure with a short course of an antibiotic. Although the risk of infection following an HSG is low, approximately 1 to 3 percent, it's important to protect your reproductive tract against any possible contamination by bacteria. In fact, if you have a history of pelvic inflammatory disease, an HSG may not be recommended and a laparoscopy might be substituted.

Although an HSG can be very painful, in the hands of a practitioner who routinely performs it (several times a month) you will probably experience only a moderate amount of discomfort. If you have a low threshold of pain, however, or are anxious about such procedures, it may be helpful to take diazepam (Valium) and an analgesic such as 600 to 800 mg of ibuprofen (Motrin, Advil) forty-five to sixty minutes beforehand. The ibuprofen will ease any pain, and the diazepam will help relax you and the muscles of your uterus and tubes, averting much of the discomfort that might occur. If you have learned or are learning relaxation techniques, practicing such a technique before, during, and after this and other procedures can be very helpful in reducing discomfort. Listening to a favorite relaxation tape may also be a help; portable tape players with headphones are inexpensive and available in many stores.

In addition to its diagnostic capability, for some women, the HSG may be therapeutic. About 30 percent of those who have a normal HSG conceive within the next six months.

Laparoscopy

Laparoscopy is a surgical procedure that utilizes two or three tiny (each is about a half inch) incisions in the abdomen. One usually is made near the navel; if others are needed, they're placed just above the pubic hairline. An extremely slender viewing instrument, the laparoscope, is inserted through the first incision in order to view the organs of the pelvic area, including the exterior of the fallopian tubes and the uterus. The laparoscope allows the surgeon to see whether the tubes look normal and whether fimbria are present and moving. The shape and outward appearance of a tube can indicate the presence of disease or obstruction. Inflammation and scarring elsewhere in the tube also may change its outward appearance. In addition, the presence and extent of endometriosis and any adhesions can be evaluated.

Laparoscopy

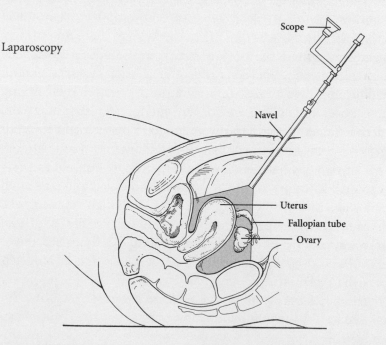

During this surgical procedure, carbon dioxide gas is pumped into the abdomen just below the navel to expand the abdominal cavity. The laparoscope is inserted through another incision to view the internal organs. Instruments can be combined with the scope to treat infertility and other gynecological problems and to remove eggs for in vitro fertilization.

Laparoscopy almost always requires general anesthesia. To provide a clearer view, carbon dioxide is injected into the abdomen to push the abdominal wall and intestines away from the reproductive organs. A short, narrow tube, a trocar, is placed in each incision to serve as a port of entry for the scope and other instruments. A light on the scope illuminates the field of view. If necessary, surgery can be performed during the laparoscopy—adhesions can be separated for a better diagnosis, misplaced endometrial tissue can be removed, and tissue samples can be taken. Such surgery may be done through a single incision, in conjunction with the scope, or it may require a second small incision.

Before the trocar is removed at the completion of this surgery, the carbon dioxide is allowed to escape and most of it does. The rest is gradually absorbed by the body. Any gas that remains may migrate upward and cause a pain near your shoulder. A small bandage will cover the incision, and after a brief recovery period, you'll be able to go home. You may want to wear relaxed clothing with a loose waistband to the hospital and for a few days afterward to accommodate a temporarily expanded waistline and to avoid aggravating any abdominal discomfort. How soon you'll want to go back to work will depend on the demands of your job. You may feel some discomfort for the next two or three days and it's a good idea to take it easy for as long as a week. Although you might be able to schedule a laparoscopy for a Thursday or Friday so that you can recover over the weekend, you should still be prepared to feel much more tired than usual for a number of days as a side effect of the anesthesia.

In the past, laparoscopy was considered a routine test, but today it is used chiefly on an individual basis, after you and your physician have weighed its risks versus its benefits. Indications for this surgical procedure include a history of pelvic infection, an abnormal HSG, symptoms that suggest endometriosis, or unexplained infertility.

Hysteroscopy

This procedure can be used instead of a hysterosalpingogram to evaluate the uterus for fibroids, polyps, or scar tissue. It's not a good test for evaluating the fallopian tubes. A hysteroscope is a slender telescopic instrument like the laparoscope, but it's inserted into your uterus by way of your cervix. It provides a good view of the uterus interior and the opening of the fallopian tubes, but does cause cramping or pain. In some instances, your physician may recommend that a hysteroscopy be performed at the same time as a laparoscopy for a more thorough examination. No anesthesia is needed for a hysteroscopy alone; if both procedures are done, however, general anesthesia is necessary.

REPAIRING TUBAL DAMAGE

Whether fallopian tubes can be surgically repaired successfully depends upon the extent and characteristics of the damage. The chance of success is poor if the tube is swollen so its diameter is more than four-fifths of an inch, there are no visible fimbria, and there are dense pelvic and ovarian adhesions. The woman's age and the duration of her infertility also affect the chance of success. Furthermore, when tubal surgery is successful and leads to pregnancy, there's a substantial risk that the embryo may implant in the tube (ectopic pregnancy). As you know, tubal pregnancies will rupture if they are not recognized and removed, and the resulting loss of blood can be life-threatening.

In many instances, treatment with in vitro fertilization (IVF) is much more successful than surgery. Although some couples will choose surgery if it's covered by their insurance and IVF is not, they should remember that not only is the success rate low, but also surgery usually must be a one-time effort because adhesions and tubal blockages generally recur—and may be worse—after each operation. *Before deciding on surgery of any substance, it's wise to get a second opinion.*

Repairing the Far End of the Tube

Surgery to repair a tubal problem is most successful if the problem is located in the far, or distal, end of the tube because this is where its diameter is greatest.

Fimbria sometimes can be restored to normal function by removing adhesions that prevent them from moving properly and by separating fimbria that are stuck together. If the opening is obstructed by adhesions, it may be possible to reopen it by dilating it. Both these corrections can be accomplished by a procedure called fimbrioplasty. If the tube's natural opening can't be restored, it may be possible to create a new opening. These procedures are performed via laparoscopy.

The success rate for such repair depends on the severity of the problem, the age of the woman, whether ovarian adhesions are present to prevent an egg from entering the fallopian tube, and other fertility factors. If the problem is severe, a study shows that after forty-eight months, the pregnancy rate is about 25 percent.

Repairing Tubal Blockages Near the Uterus

If an HSG indicates a blockage in the area where the uterus and fallopian tube are joined, a laparoscopy may be necessary to determine whether or not there's a true occlusion. If the obstruction is caused by accumulated cell debris rather than actual tissue destruction, surgery may not be needed to correct it. A technique that uses flexible-tip wire guides enables surgeons to maneuver a catheter through the uterus and into the tube. The catheter holds a small balloon that is inflated to dilate and open the blockage. In a study of this procedure, experienced practitioners achieved an open tube in a substantial percentage of women who had this sort of tubal blockage near the uterus. Twelve months after treatment, the pregnancy rate was 39 percent, of which 13 percent were ectopic pregnancies.

Rebuilding a Blocked Fallopian Tube

If your fallopian tubes are not open because of tissue damage, a skillful, experienced microsurgeon may be able to remove the damaged section and then attach what remains of the tube to your uterus. Such an operation can be performed via a conventional surgical incision (a laparotomy), which requires a longer recuperation, or with laparoscopy. This type of tubal repair is rarely successful, however, except when it's used to reverse a tubal ligation, when tubes are clipped shut or severed for birth control purposes.

If the problem is a hydrosalpinx, a fallopian tube that's fluid-filled and swollen because its far end is blocked, the success rate of treatment is not great and depends largely on the size of the hydrosalpinx and how badly the tube is injured. If the hydrosalpinx is not very large and the tubal lining is still present, it may be possible to reopen the far end of the tube or form a new opening, allowing it to drain. The chance of conceiving after this repair is about 25 percent, with a risk of ectopic pregnancy that ranges from 15 to 50 percent.

Reversing Sterilization

Reconnecting fallopian tubes that have been closed off surgically to prevent pregnancy is one of the more successful tubal repair procedures—when performed by a surgeon experienced in this procedure. The success of the repair also depends a great deal on how much of the tube remained intact after the sterilization and what part of the tube was "tied." If the middle section was severed or closed off by a clip and at least four or five centimeters (1.5 to 2 inches) of tube remain, chances of a pregnancy afterward range from 50 to 80 percent. Other factors in the success of this surgery are whether the woman is under age forty and whether the tubes have been damaged by inflammation or other conditions. This repair increasingly is performed as a laparoscopy.

THE CERVIX THAT DOESN'T PERFORM

Your cervix is an active participant in shepherding sperm from the vagina into your upper reproductive tract. During your fertile period a normal cervix secretes mucus that is thin, slippery, stretchy, and able to protect the sperm from the normally acidic vaginal fluids. An inborn malformation or trauma to its mucus-producing cells can impair the ability of the cervix to produce fertile-type mucus, making it difficult or impossible for sperm to get through it in order to enter the uterus.

Cervical Trauma

Cervical trauma can result from simple surgical procedures such as a dilation and curettage (D&C), abortion, or treatment for abnormal cells found in a Pap smear. These can injure the mucus-producing cells or the cervical tissue, and if much scarring occurs, the cervix may become stiff and narrow. If your cervix is not functioning properly because this has happened, it may be returned to normal by being stretched gently.

Hormonal Causes

Fertile-type mucus is produced by the cervical glands in response to the rise in estrogen that takes place just before ovulation. If your cervix hasn't been injured and has no structural abnormalities, the problem of nonexistent or insufficient amounts of fertile mucus might be due to a lack of estrogen receptors in the cells or to the need of those receptors for a bigger boost of estrogen to trigger mucus secretion—it's theorized that some receptors can have a higher estrogen threshold.

Hormone Treatment for Cervical Problems

If there's no obvious physical explanation for your lack of mucus secretion, and your medical history indicates that you may not be ovulating normally, using hormonal drugs to improve your ovulatory cycle may also increase your mucus production. As egg follicles enlarge in response to FSH stimulation, they secrete estrogen that usually stimulates the cervix. If the cervical cells need a small estrogen boost in order to work, improving your ovulation may also improve the production of fertile mucus.

On the negative side, however, if clomiphene therapy is used to improve your ovulation, it may directly cause the cervix to secrete nonfertile mucus. Such mucus is thick, opaque, and sticky and blocks sperm from passing into the uterus.

Intrauterine Insemination (IUI)

If neither surgery nor hormonal treatment is successful in restoring your cervix to normal functioning, it's possible to bypass the cervix by delivering your partner's sperm directly into your uterus via intrauterine insemination. IUI is used most often when a sperm count is low, or when the causes of infertility are not precisely known.

The current IUI technique requires the male to produce a semen sample a few hours before the insemination. The sample is "washed," which means the sperm is separated from the semen and concentrated. This concentrate is injected via a catheter that's threaded into your uterus, a procedure that's similar to having a Pap smear.

Most fertility centers perform IUI once or twice during each cycle. The first insemination usually takes place just before your anticipated time of ovulation and the second twenty-four hours later. You can use an ovulation test kit so that you'll know when your LH surge is occurring and about to trigger ovulation. Occasionally ultrasound may be used to see whether a follicle has been emptied or is still waiting to release an egg.

IUI is only somewhat successful. If a woman with cervical factor infertility is under age forty, IUI ordinarily results in a pregnancy rate of 3 to 7 percent per cycle. Four to six cycles produce a conception rate of about 10 to 25 percent. For women over age forty, however, the success rate is about half that. For couples with unexplained infertility or male factor infertility, the pregnancy rate is even lower: 2 to 5 percent per cycle.

However, the results of four approaches to assisted insemination—intracervical insemination alone, intrauterine insemination alone, or these two methods combined with superovulation (ovulation stimulated with gonadotropin drugs)—recently found that the highest pregnancy rate (33 percent) was achieved with a combination of IUI and gonadotropin superovulation. Treatment was given for four cycles unless pregnancy was achieved. Poorest results (10 percent) occurred in the couples who received only intracervical insemination. The other two methods—IUI alone and superovulation plus intracervical insemination—resulted in pregnancy rates of 18 and 19 percent, respectively, after four cycles. There were just over 230 couples in each treatment group.

ANDREA'S STORY

When we decided to have a second child a few years after we'd had our first, my husband and I found that we had to deal with secondary infertility. I'd had no problem becoming pregnant with our first child but now, after several miscarriages, we were faced with deciding whether or not we wanted to try infertility treatments and how far we wanted to go with them. After my third pregnancy failed, we just took some time off to think about what we would do next—if anything. Mostly we needed to understand what we were trying to communicate to each other.

Because of my age—I was thirty-six by this time—we had gone to a fertility specialist. Laparoscopy confirmed that I had endometriosis, with substantial cysts on my ovaries. I got pregnant after the surgery but I also lost that baby. I was ready to give up. I never wanted to go past a certain point in trying to have a baby. I didn't want to try fertility drugs or IVF or anything that meant we were going beyond getting pregnant chiefly by ourselves. We also were worried about having more than one baby. Neither of us wanted our lives to be as disrupted and hectic as they would be if we had two or more babies!

I was ready to think about adopting but I found that my husband has very strong feelings against adoption, that he wanted a child who was genetically his. When the doctor suggested we try IUI, I wasn't interested, but my husband thought we should—you can see there was a lot of back and forth in our discussions and our thinking about what to do and how far to go! We did try IUI and it was successful. We were lucky—we took the easier route and it worked out.

IUI is a relatively low-tech and inexpensive approach to try before you go on to more expensive assisted reproductive technologies. Each cycle of IUI alone will cost approximately $500; the addition of superovulation adds about $1300 per cycle. For the best results, it's wise to ask your physician or fertility center what their own rate of success is with these techniques.

THE IRREGULAR UTERUS

Like the fallopian tubes and the cervix, the uterus may have flaws in its structure or in its ability to function that interfere with its capacity to receive an embryo and nurture it to term.

The Non-normal Shape

The uterus is formed between the tenth and sixteenth weeks of fetal development when two tubal systems, the Müllerian ducts, broaden and join into a single structure that becomes the uterus. If this process is not fully completed, a girl may be born with a divided uterus, or two separate ones, or none at all. Of these comparatively rare occurrences, the most commonly seen forms are a uterus that is divided by a thin sheet of fibrous tissue (a septate uterus) and one that's separated by a muscular wall (a bicornuate uterus). These usually have a single cervix and each side has a fallopian tube.

Another congenital abnormality may have been caused in utero by diethylstilbestrol (DES) if this drug was taken during the first twelve to sixteen weeks of pregnancy to prevent miscarriage. In some instances, such exposure would cause a female fetus to develop a very long cervix and a very small uterine cavity. If the abnormal T-shape of the DES uterus is quite pronounced, carrying a pregnancy to term can become extremely difficult. If the irregularity is not severe, pregnancy is possible, although the lack of room in the uterine cavity makes prematurity very likely. Since DES was last used to avert miscarriage in 1971, this condition is not common.

A Bicornuate Uterus

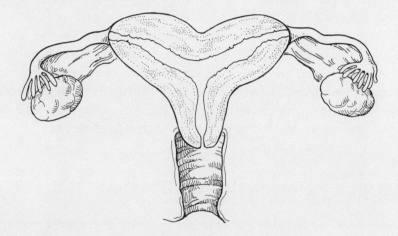

The Congenitally Abnormal Uterus and Pregnancy

Severe congenital abnormalities (which are unusual) cannot be corrected and don't permit pregnancy either to occur or to be carried to term. When the shape of the uterus is not markedly abnormal, however, a successful pregnancy may be possible. Each woman must be treated individually by a physician who is very experienced in such problems.

If your uterus is divided by a thin fibrous wall (septum) that has no blood supply or nerves, the wall can be removed more easily than a muscular division, which requires more extensive surgery. A divided uterus ordinarily is found during an HSG examination, and the type of division is confirmed with magnetic resonance imaging (MRI) or laparoscopy, although ultrasound sometimes can reveal whether the wall is a septum or is made of muscle tissue. If the partition is muscle, it's visible on the outside of the uterus during a laparoscopy.

Sometimes a split uterus can maintain a pregnancy to term with the partition intact and sometimes it cannot. Although there's no good data on this, the risk of miscarriage appears to be higher, especially if the uterus is divided by a septum.

As you can imagine, these are high-risk pregnancies that usually introduce a number of practical problems into a couple's life. Before a woman with an irregular uterus tries to conceive, she probably should discuss very thoroughly with her physician all the risks and possible difficulties that may occur, such as miscarriage, premature labor, and perhaps a complicated delivery.

Common, Nonstructural Uterine Problems

Most of the uterine abnormalities that a woman may experience are not inborn; instead, they generally develop during her reproductive years. Most common are fibroids and Asherman's syndrome, with fibroids being the single most frequently seen uterine problem.

Fibroids

These benign tumors of smooth muscle tissue grow slowly in the inner or outer layers of the muscular wall or protrude from the wall into the cavity of the uterus. They can be as small as a pea or become as large as a grapefruit, although most are between a walnut and an orange in size. Fibroids affect at least 20 to 40 percent of most women by the time they're in their thirties and forties. However, almost 50 percent of African-American women are likely to have them. Fibroids run in families, although the cause is not known.

A substantial proportion of fibroids cause no symptoms, but when they do, the symptom frequently is excessive vaginal bleeding; fibroid location usually determines the type of symptom. *Submucosal fibroids,* those growing just under the endometrium, are a common cause of heavy bleeding that occurs chiefly during menstrual periods and occasionally at other times. Submucosal fibroids that eventually protrude into the uterine cavity may cause cramps as the uterus tries to get rid of them. *Intramural fibroids,* those growing in the muscle layers of the uterus, can cause pain and other problems if they press against nerves, the bladder, or the bowel. A fibroid can block a fallopian tube or cause miscarriage if it presses on the cervix.

Submucosal fibroids are a fertility hazard because they cause the uterus to react as it would to any foreign body. They can disturb the normal development of the endometrium and interfere

Uterine Fibroids

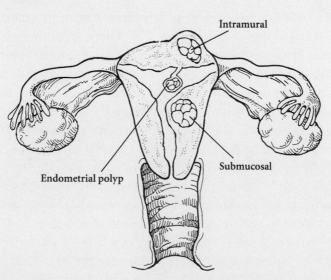

with other changes that need to take place to prepare the uterus for an embryo. Large fibroids also can distort the uterus enough to cause recurrent miscarriage. Or they may compress blood vessels and reduce blood flow to the fetus. They also grow rapidly during pregnancy, crowding the fetus and increasing the risk of a premature delivery.

DIAGNOSING AND TREATING FIBROIDS. Fibroids may be suspected during a pelvic exam if your uterus feels irregular or unusually large. Ultrasound is commonly used to determine their size and location. If the fibroids are within your uterus, they're removed through the cervical canal and vagina with the help of a hysteroscope, under anesthesia. The scope enables a surgeon to see into the uterus, use a wire loop or laser to cut out the fibroids, and then heat-seal the endometrium. The danger of damaging the uterine muscle or endometrium during this procedure is low.

If fibroids are on the outside of the uterus, they're reached through a conventional abdominal incision or by laparoscopy and removed from the uterine wall one by one, a procedure called a myomectomy. A woman who conceives after a myomectomy is likely to need a cesarean section if the uterus had to be cut open completely. Nevertheless, a myomectomy is not a hysterectomy—it removes the fibroids but leaves the uterus. Like all operations, it should be performed by a surgeon who does a lot of them and whose goal is to preserve or reestablish your reproductive capability. If you've been told that your fibroids are so large or so numerous that you must have a hysterectomy, it would be very wise to get a second opinion.

Fibroid embolization, a new approach to treating fibroids, particularly those that are numerous or deeply embedded in the uterus, looks promising because it shrinks the tumors by blocking their blood supply. At this time, however, it appears that 1 to 2 percent of women may require an emergency hysterectomy after being treated with this technique because of uterine damage. Because of this risk, and potential permanent damage to the uterus, fibroid embolization is not recommended for women who hope to become pregnant.

Asherman's Syndrome

This refers to scar tissue that can form in the uterus and interfere with the endometrium's normal cycle of development. It might occur after a miscarriage, postpartum bleeding, abnormal bleeding, an abortion, or after a cesarean section. Scarring often follows surgical procedures and, in the uterus, might range from a few scars to cases so severe the entire cavity is a mass of scar tissue. If you've had one of these events and you're ovulating but not menstruating, it may be because you have little or no functioning endometrium left.

REPAIRING ASHERMAN'S SYNDROME. As you can imagine, removing scar tissue from within the uterus is a delicate and difficult job. If you have a mild case of Asherman's, this surgery can be done via the hysteroscope, under anesthesia. Microscissors are used to snip away each scar. Afterward, you are likely to be prescribed high doses of estrogen for a month, in order to encourage the growth of whatever endometrial tissue exists so that you might again have a functioning uterine lining.

In severe cases of this syndrome, the scar tissue grows from one side of the uterus to the other, frequently binding the sides together. Not surprisingly, this circumstance demands very delicate surgery and the skills of an experienced practitioner because it's difficult to tell where scar tissue ends and the wall of the uterus begins. Couples need to realize that scar tissue often regrows after this repair. Furthermore, the interior of the uterus may be so badly damaged by scar tissue that there's not even enough endometrial tissue left to regenerate. Without a functioning endometrium, pregnancy will not take place.

ENDOMETRIOSIS AND INFERTILITY

Endometriosis occurs when endometrial tissue migrates from the uterus, probably exiting from the far end of the fallopian tubes during menstruation, implants itself elsewhere in the pelvic cavity, and grows. This tissue frequently can be found growing on the ovaries, the tubes, the bladder, the bowel, the outside of the uterus, and on the ligaments that support the uterus—almost anywhere, in fact. No matter where it implants, endometrial tissue often remains under the influence of a woman's monthly hormonal cycle and sheds cells and blood at the end of the cycle. In addition, the presence of such misplaced tissue can result in chronic inflammation and the development of scar tissue.

Endometriosis

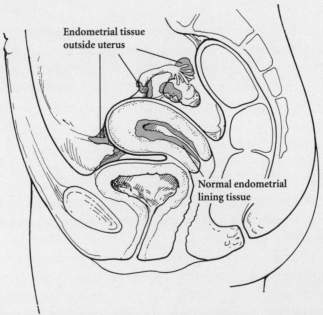

Side view of the female reproductive tract showing the presence of endometrial tissue.

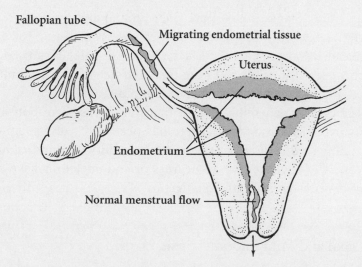

Front view of the reproductive tract showing endometrial tissue migrating through the fallopian tube.

The symptoms of endometriosis vary and reflect the location of the endometrial tissue, not its extent. They may include severe menstrual discomfort, pain during intercourse, backache, abdominal pains, discomfort during bowel movements, diarrhea, and constipation. Symptoms often are worse during menstruation.

Because even one bit of tissue will incite inflammation throughout the pelvic area, even mild endometriosis may be associated with infertility. A chronic disease that can last until menopause, endometriosis is most often diagnosed when a woman is in her twenties or thirties as part of an infertility workup or because she's experiencing pelvic pain.

For treatment purposes, the American Society for Reproductive Medicine has advocated dividing the extent of this disease into four stages. Stages III and IV endometriosis are the moderate and severe cases, and include women with major pelvic adhesions that injure and cover the surface of the ovaries and distort the fallopian tubes. Stages I and II are the minimal and mild cases, in which the patches of misplaced tissue can be as small as the size of a pinhead or a pea. The disease is diagnosed through laparoscopy, which makes it possible to locate the endometrial tissue, remove it, and, if possible, restore the pelvic anatomy to normal.

Although it's generally thought that this disease is responsible for many cases of infertility, there has been some disagreement about how badly mild cases might affect fertility. Most reproductive specialists believe that all degrees of endometriosis have the capability of negatively affecting fertility.

Minimal and Mild Endometriosis

The deposits of aberrant tissue in stages I and II endometriosis usually are too small and too few to affect the anatomy of the tubes or ovaries, yet a woman with this slight degree of disease may still have difficulty getting pregnant. A number of researchers now suspect that a mild form could cause a functional abnormality. A woman with early stage endometriosis might have more than the normal amount of fluid in her pelvis and it may contain increased levels of white blood cells, probably as a reaction to the presence of the endometrial tissue. Some women with early stage endometriosis have a luteal phase problem, abnormal follicle growth or luteinized follicles that don't rupture, or multiple and premature surges of luteinizing hormone. All of these may contribute to infertility.

Although many reproductive specialists still feel that surgical treatment of mild forms of this disease is not likely to improve fertility, several recent studies demonstrate that surgical treatment of stages I and II endometriosis can improve a woman's chance of conceiving.

In one study, infertile women with mild disease were treated with either diagnostic laparoscopy alone or with laparoscopy plus destruction of the endometriosis tissue. Those who had laparoscopy to destroy the misplaced endometrial tissue were almost twice as likely to conceive in the following nine months as a matched group of women who had only diagnostic laparoscopy.

In other research, infertile women with early endometriosis were randomized into four groups receiving one of four levels of treatment: no treatment, clomiphene alone, clomiphene plus human menopausal gonadotropin, or IVF. It was found that each of these levels of treatment increased their chances of becoming pregnant, with IVF producing the most pregnancies.

Although these recent small studies still need to be verified by research on more women with this problem, the results imply that treating even early stage endometriosis with surgery or ovulation-stimulating hormones can improve fertility.

Moderate to Severe Endometriosis

For the woman who has stage III or IV endometriosis, a number of studies have shown that removing the misplaced tissue and adhesions can improve her ability to conceive. The rate of pregnancy is highest in the six to twelve months immediately after such surgery. If pregnancy doesn't occur, however, additional surgery isn't useful. Instead, follow-up hormone therapy—with or without IUI— may lead to pregnancy if the fallopian tubes are open. If it doesn't, IVF is your best option.

It's worth mentioning that surgery for endometriosis may cost as much as one cycle of IVF, and achieving a pregnancy after surgery is likely to take longer than becoming pregnant via IVF, which can be a concern for some women. Nevertheless, many couples and their physicians prefer to try surgery first, while others will choose to go directly to IVF.

The majority of infertile couples with inborn or developed anatomical problems, and their doctors, opt for the same staircase approach to infertility treatment that we describe in Step 5. The steps include: (1 & 2) identifying and correcting all infertility factors; (3) using clomiphene alone, with other drugs, or with IUI; (4) gonadotropin therapy with or without IUI; and (5) assisted reproductive technologies—usually IVF.

The choice of treatment is affected by many factors, particularly by the type of anatomical problem involved and whether the sperm count is low. The lower the sperm count, the lower the likelihood that IUI will be helpful. Other things to consider are how much time each treatment may require, whether the woman has a strong negative reaction to hormone drugs, how long it might take afterward to become pregnant, and which treatments are covered by the couple's health insurance. For women over age thirty-five, the first three steps should be completed as rapidly as possible; women who are under age thirty can spend more time on those phases of treatment. It is always a good idea to get a second opinion before starting treatment.

QUESTIONS TO ASK YOUR DOCTOR

- ⋄ Are there options other than surgery that are available?

- ⋄ Why do you recommend this particular procedure?

- ⋄ How often do you perform this procedure?

- ⋄ Will you explain what happens before and during it?

- ⋄ If I am anxious about having this, what medication can I use?

- ⋄ How soon will I be able to go back to work, especially if my job requires a lot of walking? How soon will I be able to travel?

- ⋄ What sort of pain relief will I have available if I need it afterward?

- ⋄ What are the success rates of the options that are most feasible for me?

- ⋄ What are their costs?

Step 6B:
Diagnose and Treat Male Problems

Until recent years there weren't many treatments for the disorders that prevent some men from becoming biological fathers. More progress is being made now, however, and men who have what is called male factor infertility today have a greater chance than ever to father their own biological children. Microsurgery, hormone treatments, and assisted reproductive technologies are available to overcome a variety of male infertility disorders.

Unlike female factor infertility, male factor problems do not lend themselves to a many-step treatment approach. A medical history and physical usually turn up 95 percent of the possible problems that could be contributing to or causing a couple's infertility. At this point, the choices are few: the cause is either treatable or not. If it's not, the only alternative generally is an assisted reproductive technology.

For about 25 percent of infertile couples, male factor problems—sperm that are sparse in number, malformed, or somehow lacking in fertilizing ability—either may be the sole reason or a contributing factor. If your semen tests have been persistently abnormal, you may want to see a urologist who has had special training in diagnosing and working with male infertility, a branch of medicine called andrology. In the past, when couples couldn't conceive, the male partner frequently wasn't examined until the woman had gone through extensive testing. Today, we recommend that both of you be tested simultaneously in order to save time and because it would not be unusual for each of you to have a fertility problem.

Many fertility centers have an andrologist on staff or may be able to refer you to one. If you want to interview more than one specialist—always a good idea—RESOLVE is also an excellent source for referrals. Local RESOLVE chapters are listed in the business section of the white pages of your telephone directory; if you can't find a local chapter, call the national office at 617-623-0744 for information about referrals to reproductive specialists. Furthermore, the guidelines we suggest in Step 5, pages 148–149, for selecting a reproductive endocrinologist also apply to choosing a urologist or andrologist. You not only want to find a physician with extensive experience in this field, you also want someone with whom you are at ease, who communicates well, and who will make you feel as comfortable as possible through the testing and treatment process.

FINDING THE PROBLEM

It's important that the physician you choose takes a detailed health history. Don't be surprised if you are asked about how frequently and when during your partner's menstrual cycle you have intercourse. Physicians have learned that even sophisticated couples may not be clear about when ovulation occurs or how long sperm live. Simply having intercourse more frequently around the time of ovulation can lead to pregnancy in couples who feared they were infertile.

One of the first things couples are asked to do during infertility workups is to find out when the woman is ovulating, because having intercourse more frequently during ovulation, and one or two days before it, sometimes can be surprisingly helpful in resolving infertility. (The sketch of the menstrual cycle in Step 2, page 49, illustrates how the ovulatory or fertile period is approximately five days of the menstrual cycle.)

In actual practice, it's all right to have intercourse as often as you'd like around ovulation, and if you're not in the mood, well, we remind our patients that "there's always tomorrow." You want to remember that the most important thing here is to sustain your relationship as a couple and not let anxiety about infertility rule your lives.

Because sperm can survive about two days in the vagina when the cervical mucus is hospitable, it's generally thought that it's most effective to have intercourse at least every other day during a woman's fertile time. Just how often, however, hasn't been determined. No scientific findings support the conventional recommendation that intercourse every other day is more likely to result in conception than having intercourse every day. In fact, recent evidence suggests that optimal timing can vary from couple to couple.

In addition to taking your health history, your physician will give you a thorough physical exam aimed at finding possible abnormalities of the testicles or prostate or whether veins in the scrotum might be unusually dilated, a condition called a varicocele that can lead to male infertility.

In all likelihood, the specialist who examines you also will want to have another set of sperm tests made because there can be variations from one sperm sample to another and from one lab to another. In addition, an analysis of certain hormone levels in your blood can supply clues to the health of your testicles. It's important to realize that a sperm analysis will reveal the volume of semen, the number of sperm (20 million plus per cubic centimeter of semen is considered normal), the percentage of motile (able to move) sperm (the norm is 50 percent or more), and the percentage of sperm with normal shapes (the norm varies from lab to lab). The analysis is not able to measure how well your sperm can function. If any one of these parameters is abnormal, the analysis should be repeated four to six weeks later.

If the new lab tests reveal few or no sperm, your physician may suggest that a biopsy be made of your testicular tissue to determine what is going on at the testicular level. When FSH is markedly elevated, it suggests that the testicles are making few or no sperm. A biopsy also can help your physician determine whether you have a tubal blockage, which could be treatable, or a serious abnormality of the sperm-generating tissues, which can't be corrected.

A biopsy generally can be performed with local, spinal, or general anesthesia, depending on the patient's wishes. A tiny (1 to 2 cm) incision is made through the skin of the scrotum and the testes and a small amount of tissue is removed for study. The tissue is examined under the microscope for evidence of sperm production. Sometimes the tissue looks as if it's functioning normally, and the problem lies elsewhere—in the ducts that transport the sperm.

The incision is closed with an absorbable suture. Complications are infrequent, the most common being some bleeding. The procedure takes about thirty minutes and most men return to work after a day of taking it easy. There's some mild pain afterward that can be alleviated with ibuprofen.

Your medical history, physical examination, and the tests will uncover almost all of the possible causes of infertility: erectile dysfunction (impotence), a structural problem, a hormonal imbalance, a genetic disorder, or a cause that can't be found with current technology. It is always a good idea to get a second opinion after a diagnosis is made. Simply request copies of your record and test results for the purpose of consultation.

ERECTILE DYSFUNCTION

Erectile dysfunction, once known as impotence, is a common problem. It's defined as the inability to have an erection that's adequate for intercourse more than one-fourth of the time. Traditionally, impotence generally was associated with aging, and about 2 percent of all forty-year-olds were thought to have this problem, with the number increasing with age. However, a 1998 study by researchers at the University of Chicago and the Robert Wood Johnson Medical School reports that erectile dysfunction today appears to occur more frequently in younger men than was thought. The researchers found that 7 percent of men aged eighteen to twenty-nine and 9 percent of men in their thirties, for example, could not have or maintain an erection. Impotence was experienced with increasing frequency after age forty.

Causes

Until fifteen or twenty years ago it was believed that most cases of erectile dysfunction were psychologically caused; today, however, it's known that most impotence has a physical source; as a result, a variety of treatments are now available. The ability to have an erection depends on a healthy blood supply to the penis, and treatments are designed to increase and hold this blood flow. The erectile tissue of the penis contains a network of blood vessels controlled by the spinal nerves. During arousal the vessels enlarge, more blood flows into the penis, and it stiffens. Muscle tissue tightens to hold the blood in place so that the erection is maintained.

Anything that damages a man's blood circulation or his spinal nerves can cause this system to fail. Diabetes mellitus, atherosclerosis (fatty deposits in the arteries), and spinal injuries can cause impotence. Lack of exercise, poor nutrition, and a high alcohol intake may contribute to it. Certain medications, particularly some of the drugs used to treat hypertension, also can affect blood flow.

Only about 15 percent of the time is impotence due to psychological problems such as stress, depression, or interpersonal problems. Almost all men find it impossible to achieve or maintain an erection at some time. The ability to have an erection can be highly variable, depending on a man's physical health and state of mind. Like many health issues, if impotence occurs so often it becomes a problem, it's probably more useful to do something about it rather than just worry.

Treatments

The first treatment option is to avoid or stop any activity that might injure the circulatory or nervous system and lead to impotence: using alcohol, cocaine, or cigarettes, and taking long bike rides, especially on hard, narrow bicycle seats that compress penile blood vessels. If you or your doctor suspects that a prescription drug may be the cause, it may be possible to find an alternative. But only doctors should change prescription medications.

Furthermore, when it comes to your testicles, keep them cool. The sperm-producing capability of the testes can be impaired if they're kept just a few degrees warmer than their normal temperature of 96 degrees Fahrenheit. And, as we mentioned in Step 1, it's a good idea to avoid hot baths, saunas, and tight pants or bicycle shorts.

Medical treatments that are available include:

Sildenafil (Viagra), a prescription chemical in pill form that increases the amount of guanosine monophosphate (GMP) in the body. GMP is what makes blood vessels expand, and its production usually is triggered naturally when a man becomes aroused. Sildenafil increases GMP by inhibiting the enzyme that inactivates it.

Sildenafil helps most men have an erection, even if the cause is psychological. It should be noted, however, that this pill doesn't work in every man who uses it, nor does it always lead to erections that are sufficient for intercourse. This medication works only if a man is sexually aroused; it doesn't increase desire.

Sildenafil doesn't appear to improve erections in men whose impotence is caused by uncontrolled diabetes or alcohol abuse. Side effects include headaches, flushing, and gastrointestinal upset in 20 to 30 percent of those who use it. Up to 10 percent of users experience temporary disturbances in their color vision at the customary doses of 50 to 100 mg.

Fatalities have occurred with this drug in men who had very low or very high blood pressure, or had a recent heart attack, or were on medications such as nitroglycerin (a nitrate drug) and propranolol for heart disease. Sildenafil's action is not limited to the penis; it affects the entire body and, when combined with nitrate drugs, can cause sudden severe drops in blood pressure. The long-term effects of this impotence drug are not yet known.

Alprostadil is another drug that increases blood flow to the penis. However, because it's not absorbed into the blood in substantial amounts it's less likely than sildenafil to produce side effects. Alprostadil isn't taken orally, but is injected with a very fine needle into the base of the penis or, as a soft pellet about the size of a grain of rice, it's put inside the opening of the penis. About 90 percent of the time, an application of alprostadil causes an erection sufficient for intercourse. This drug takes about twenty minutes to work and you don't have to be aroused. If you choose alprostadil to treat your erectile dysfunction, you'll probably get the first injection in the doctor's office so that the dose can be adjusted and you can learn to inject it yourself.

The most common side effect of this method is a modest amount of discomfort at the site of the injection. In some men this drug has caused uncomfortably prolonged erections (priapism) that require a shot of epinephrine to reverse. Reversal treatment—from a doctor or an emergency room—needs to be given quite promptly to avoid permanent damage to penile tissue. Prolonged erections and discomfort at the injection site aren't problems when alprostadil pellets are slipped into the opening of the penis. Other side effects are rare and men who are taking nitrate drugs also can use alprostadil.

Testosterone therapy can be effective for men whose levels of this hormone are unusually low. It can be administered via injection or a skin patch. This should be used only in men with documented low serum testosterone. Because it carries a slight risk of stimulating an indolent prostate cancer, it should be taken only under the guidance of an andrologist or urologist who is knowledgeable about its effects.

Psychotherapy—often for both partners—may prove helpful when the cause of impotence does not appear to be physical. Therapy usually focuses on improving attitudes toward sex, exploring troublesome inhibitions or past traumas, and improving communication between sexual partners.

A *vacuum pump* can be used to produce an erection without drugs. The pump is a clear plastic cylinder that fits over the penis and is activated by hand to create a partial vacuum, pulling blood into the penis. A tension ring tightened around the base of the penis traps the blood to maintain the erection. Possible side effects can be discomfort or pain, numbness, and bruising.

ABNORMAL ANATOMY

A variety of structural abnormalities—some congenital, some acquired—of the ejaculatory duct (vas deferens) and/or the fine, coiled tubes in which the sperm mature (epididymis) can interfere with the normal passage of sperm into the penis for ejaculation. For the man who wishes to become a father, these anatomical problems sometimes can be corrected with surgery.

Obstructions Due to Infection

Blockages can form in the epididymis, the narrow, coiled duct that links the testicles to the passage known as the vas deferens. When infections of the male genital tract are not treated, the result can be inflammation and scarring in this slender tube, about one and a half times the diameter of a human hair. Such damage, especially if the infection recurs or becomes chronic, may permanently block the epididymis or injure testicular tissue. Inflammation also can impair the ability of sperm to fertilize eggs, or just to be able to swim well.

Tests for infectious agents in the genital tract secretions of infertile men may reveal that bacteria and viruses are present, often without symptoms. Most genital tract infections are sexually transmitted and, if not noticed and treated, may be passed back and forth between sexual partners, causing additional inflammation and scar tissue. A nonsexually transmitted infection is mumps. If it infects boys after puberty, the testes may become inflamed in about 25 percent of the cases. In those rare instances in which it affects both testicles, this may result in sterility.

Semen quality and fertility have been found to improve in infertile men after they've been treated with antibiotics, often a combination of at least two antibiotics. This improvement, however, can take weeks to months to occur.

Obstruction of the Vas Deferens

The vas deferens is the ejaculatory duct that carries the sperm from the epididymis to the penis. It can be blocked deliberately by clips or sutures for the purpose of birth control; it can be accidentally damaged during surgery on nearby tissue; and, in rare instances, a male baby may be born without this duct. Depending on the

184 SIX STEPS TO INCREASED FERTILITY

anatomy involved, it may be possible to repair such anatomical conditions surgically, to restore sperm to the ejaculate. If this can't be done, it's usually possible to bypass the problem by collecting enough active, healthy sperm from the epididymis to use with in vitro fertilization (IVF) when a pregnancy is wanted.

Surgery to repair obstructions in the epididymis necessitates the use of powerful magnification and suture material that's one-seventh the diameter of a human hair. In the hands of a surgeon who performs such procedures often, the success rates are quite high: sperm return to the ejaculate in more than 75 percent of cases. The surgery costs about $10,000.

Connecting Egg and Sperm with ICSI

If infection control or surgery can't correct the problem of too few or no sperm in your ejaculate or sperm that won't perform, a new technique available today may make it possible to overcome this impediment to fatherhood. Intracytoplasmic sperm injection, commonly known as ICSI, is a single-sperm injection technique that makes it possible for many men, who have either very few sperm (oligospermia) or no sperm (azoospermia) in their ejaculate, to become fathers.

If sperm are present in your semen but they're too few to reach an egg via the conventional route, they can be collected from the semen. If there are no sperm in your ejaculate, a needle aspiration procedure can be used to withdraw sperm from the epididymis or testis. If this is unsuccessful, the next step is to remove a bit of the sperm-generating tissue from inside the testicle that, hopefully, will contain sperm.

A needle aspiration can take up to thirty minutes; if the urologist has to do the second step, the entire procedure may require up to one hour. It's performed under local or general anesthesia as outpatient surgery. When sperm have been retrieved, one is injected into each of the mature eggs that have been collected during IVF, and the eggs are placed in a culture to develop into embryos.

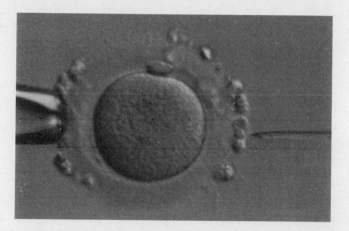

Close-up of ICSI procedure showing egg about to be injected with sperm: the egg is in the center, the holding pipette is on the left, and the injection needle is at the right.

After an aspiration procedure, you'll recover from the anesthetic fairly quickly and with few side effects, although you are likely to be sore and uncomfortable for a day or so. An ice pack will help to reduce inflammation. You'll want to avoid heavy physical activity for a week and stay away from anything strenuous, including lifting, for about a month.

With the help of ICSI, almost all men whose semen contain very few sperm, a condition called oligospermia, will have enough sperm to inject the eggs produced during an IVF cycle. And about half those who have no sperm at all in their semen will have some in their testicular tissue.

JIM'S STORY

After I had a kidney transplant some years ago, I no longer produced semen or sperm. When I married and we wanted to have children, I began seeing various medical specialists to find the cause of this and what could be done about it. My doctors were baffled. It appeared that only exploratory surgery would tell us what was wrong. But an operation was out of the question because of the danger it would pose to my transplanted kidney.

A testicular biopsy was considered safe, however, and it showed that there were sperm in the tissue. For some reason, perhaps because my vas deferens might have been damaged during the transplant, sperm were not being ejaculated. Fortunately, they could be gotten from the tissue and, with the help of ICSI and IVF, they could be injected into my wife's eggs.

My wife and I tried the combined procedure for four cycles and we had several setbacks. Suzanne reacted strongly to the drugs used to stimulate her ovaries, and too many eggs were produced. (When large numbers of eggs are ovulated, they usually aren't properly matured and don't develop well.) She also was hospitalized for ovarian hyperstimulation. On our fourth try, however, there were fewer eggs and five developed into embryos and were transferred. That's more than usual, but Suzanne was thirty-seven, an age when her embryos would be less likely to do well. We felt twins or triplets would be okay, but if it turned out that there were more, we would've thought about selective reduction. We were lucky, though. We had twins and they're just perfect.

In two recent studies, the fertilization rate for ICSI was 33 and 42 percent, respectively, for each attempt, and it's now considered the state-of-the-art technique for treating severe male factor infertility. Its pregnancy success rate, however, depends largely on the number and quality of the eggs that are fertilized this way. The cost of ICSI is about $10,000 or more.

ICSI and Genetic Disease

ICSI is not without risk. Although this technique offers some infertile men their only hope of having biologically related children, those whose lack of sperm is genetically based will probably pass on their problem to any sons they may have. A gene deletion on the Y chromosome accounts for infertility in about 10 to 15 percent of men with azoospermia. Because the presence of the Y chromosome determines the male gender, in all likelihood, male children born to men with the Y deletion will have the same infertility problem as their fathers. (Female children are not at risk because they inherit an X chromosome, not a Y, from their fathers.) This defect in the Y chromosome occurs spontaneously and, before ICSI, wasn't passed along because the men in whom it occurred could not father children.

The possibility that these genetic deletions are being transmitted to male children via ICSI is being studied by several research groups. It should be noted, however, that many boys born with this gene deletion may also be able to father children with the help of ICSI. We tell our patients about this possibility and provide them with the latest information on ICSI, and we encourage them to use it because its positive results at this time appear to outweigh future problems.

If an infertile man has normally functioning testes but no sperm in his ejaculate, there's a small (1 to 2 percent) chance that he was born without a vas deferens. This also can be overcome with ICSI. However, today it's also known that most men who are born without a vas deferens also have the gene for cystic fibrosis. Males who have this disease often die before they become adults; men who have the gene but not the disease incur the risk of passing it on when they father children if their partner also is a carrier of the gene. Some fertility centers today have the capability to test embryos for such genetic diseases before they're transferred to the uterus.

Donor Insemination

If you have azoospermia and a thorough examination has found that your partner has a healthy reproductive system, together you may want to consider using donor sperm. This approach, once termed artificial insemination, has been used frequently and successfully for many years.

Most often, the sperm is separated from the ejaculate, concentrated, and inserted into the uterus via intrauterine insemination (IUI). (IUI is described in detail in Step 6A, pages 161–164.) Sometimes the donor sperm is simply placed into the cervix during the fertile time of the woman's cycle. Separating sperm from the ejaculate, sometimes called washing sperm, can improve its performance because the process also filters normally shaped, motile sperm from abnormal, less motile sperm. Donor sperm can be used for any assisted reproductive technology procedure.

Frozen donor sperm can be obtained from sperm banks throughout the country. Because it's readily available, with the help of your fertility specialist or center you should be able to find sperm from a man who has physical and other traits that closely resemble those of your family. Donors are classified by such characteristics as race, height, weight, hair and eye color, blood group and type, age, occupation, religion, education, and nationality. Often couples have access to sperm from several donors who closely resemble the male partner, making it possible to select with some exactness the characteristics they prefer.

Today sperm banks are required to test prospective donors for antibodies to the AIDS virus and for other sexually transmitted diseases that might be passed along in the semen. Don't take for granted, however, that this safeguard is in use. Instead, obtain written information about the screening procedures from the bank you're considering.

Don't take sperm quality for granted, either, because quality control can vary significantly among sperm banks. Ask your fertility specialist for an analysis of the sperm sample that spells out the number of sperm and the percentage that appears normally shaped and active. It also may be helpful to ask about the experience that the fertility center or your specialist has had with a particular donor bank.

Don't forget, however, that the success of donor insemination will depend a great deal on the age and health of the eggs that are being fertilized. Women under age thirty-five with no female infertility factor have a pregnancy rate of 80 percent after six cycles of insemination with donor sperm. The rate for women who are over age thirty-five is 40 percent after six cycles. The cost of using donor sperm can range from $300 to $500 for each cycle.

Reversing Vasectomy

Vasectomy has long been one of the most frequently used forms of birth control. Although the men who choose this very effective method are warned that they shouldn't consider it a reversible procedure, in the hands of a very skilled surgeon the disruption of the vas deferens can be corrected through microsurgery. The success of this operation, called a vasovasostomy, depends not only on the skill of the surgeon, but also on the interval of time between the original procedure and the reversal. Furthermore, the duct on the one side may have become distended from the fluid that builds up behind the clip, while the other half has remained the same in diameter. Rejoining two disparate halves can require

some very exacting microsurgery. Vasovasostomy may be performed with a local, spinal, or general anesthetic and requires a
recovery time of one or two days. The average cost for a vasovasostomy is about $8000 to $10,000.

Hypospadias

Hypospadias is a structural abnormality in which the opening of
the urethra isn't at the tip of the penis, as it normally would be,
but instead is located under the head or shaft of the penis, perhaps
halfway down or even where the penis emerges from the scrotum.
This congenital malformation is found in approximately 5 to 10
percent of infertile men. It usually is not difficult to correct and
the surgery often is performed before a boy reaches puberty.

Sites of Hypospadias

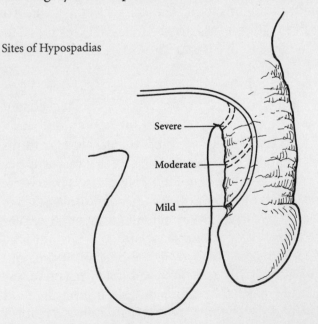

Hypospadias, showing abnormal urethral openings that might occur anywhere
underneath the shaft of the penis. Openings can vary in length.

Undescended Testicles

Undescended testicles (cryptorchidism) is an abnormality that occurs before birth. Testicles that remain in the abdomen usually don't develop properly and aren't capable of normal sperm generation. Sometimes even early surgery to move the testicles into their normal place in the scrotum may not succeed in averting later infertility. In general, surgery to correct this problem should take place before the child is eighteen to twenty-four months old.

In many instances, however, only one testicle remains in the abdomen. If only one makes the descent, fertility usually is diminished; if both remain in the abdomen, infertility almost always is the result. Undescended testicles also can increase the risk of testicular cancer later in life.

Varicocele

Another common anatomic problem that begins to be seen as boys reach adolescence is a varicocele, a painless condition in which the veins in the scrotum become enlarged just like varicose veins in the legs. The distended veins do not drain blood away from the testicles as efficiently as normal veins and blood tends to pool in the testicles, thereby raising their temperature. The testes temperature of infertile men with varicoceles has been found to be about 2 degrees Fahrenheit higher than the normal testicular temperature of fertile men without varicoceles, enough to adversely affect sperm and testosterone production.

Almost all varicoceles occur on the left side; if you have one, you may be able to feel the enlarged veins through the skin of the scrotum, especially when you're standing up.

A varicocele is found in about 15 percent of adult men; however, approximately 40 percent of men being evaluated for infertility will have it. A varicocele is suspected as a possible cause of infertility when the testes are small or when a semen analysis shows low numbers of sperm overall, large numbers of abnormally shaped sperm, or sperm that don't move vigorously.

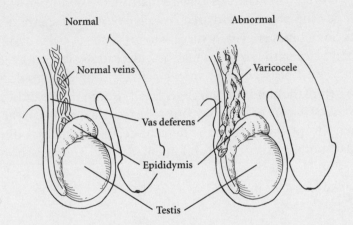

Normal testicular veins (left); varicocele (right).

Varicoceles also are associated with substantial testicular damage that may affect sperm generation and growth. Although it's not known precisely how a varicocele causes such damage, a number of studies have shown an improvement in semen and in the size and structure of the testicles after a varicocelectomy, in which the swollen veins are carefully isolated and tied off. This is delicate surgery that is performed with a variety of techniques.

Multiple surgical techniques can be used for varicocele repair. No single technique is universally used and no technique has been proved to be clearly superior. Generally speaking, after having varicocele repair, one-third of the men will achieve a conception, one-third will have greater numbers of sperm or better quality sperm in their semen analyses but will not achieve a conception, and one-third will demonstrate no benefit. At this time, it's impossible to predict beforehand which men will benefit from varicocele surgery.

However, there's another aspect to consider when trying to decide whether to have varicocele surgery. A large five-year study has found that this condition progresses over time. Even men who already have fathered children may not be able to initiate a pregnancy some years later because of sperm abnormalities resulting from a varicocele that has become more severe.

We agree with other clinicians experienced in this field that the mere presence of a varicocele in a subfertile male is not, by itself, an indication for surgical repair. Furthermore, before deciding on surgery, it's important to be certain that you have no other causes for infertility and that your partner's fertility status has been evaluated thoroughly. And, it is a good idea to seek a second opinion before committing to surgery.

Varicocele surgery is performed on an outpatient basis, using a local, spinal, or general anesthesia, depending on the patient's or surgeon's preference. For example, if an inguinal approach is used, an incision is made in the area just above the groin and the larger veins that drain blood from the testes are tied off. This area will remain sore and painful for about a week afterward, during which time the patient should avoid strenuous activity. Any analgesic like ibuprofen can be used to relieve discomfort. The cost of this procedure ranges from $6000 to $8000.

Retrograde Ejaculation

When semen goes backward into the bladder instead of being ejaculated through the penis, it's called retrograde ejaculation. Although some men are born with this condition, it's often caused by acquired disorders that affect the nerves controlling the muscles at the base (neck) of the bladder. These muscles normally close off the bladder during ejaculation. When they don't function and the neck of the bladder doesn't close, the ejaculate goes into the bladder during an orgasm. The controlling nerves may be weakened or injured by various causes: neurological disease, surgery on the neck of the bladder, prostate surgery, extensive pelvic surgery, spinal cord injury, diabetes mellitus, or the use of certain medications.

If your sperm test shows a low volume of total ejaculate, or your urine has a milky look to it, the cause may be retrograde ejaculation. The definitive test usually is a sample of urine taken immediately after an orgasm that contains lots of active sperm.

Some men with this condition respond positively to medical therapy with drugs such as ephedrine, pseudoephedrine, imipramine, and phenylpropanolamine. If these don't help the muscles of the bladder neck to function properly, sperm can be recovered from the bladder and used for intrauterine insemination.

Two methods are used to recover sperm from urine. In the simplest, four doses of oral bicarbonate (in tablet form) are taken daily for two days to neutralize the urine so that its normal acidity doesn't damage the sperm. Then urine is collected right after an ejaculation and processed to sort out the healthy sperm for IUI.

A more invasive procedure involves inserting a catheter into the bladder, rinsing out that organ, and then infusing it with a semen-protecting medium. Immediately after an ejaculation the bladder is drained either via the catheter or by urination. The healthiest sperm are recovered from the urine and used for insemination.

HORMONAL IRREGULARITIES

In a man, the hormonal signals from the hypothalamus to the nearby pituitary gland regulate the production of male sex hormones and the development of healthy sperm in the testes. If the testes are correctly performing their task of growing sperm, certain cells produce other hormones and chemicals that provide feedback to the hypothalamus and pituitary and modulate their output.

Normal sperm production depends entirely on a highly coordinated, physiologic communication and cooperation among all parts of the male reproductive system, which sometimes has to perform under unfavorable genetic and environmental conditions.

An analysis of the blood can show whether hormone levels are normal. Abnormally high amounts of follicle-stimulating hormone (FSH) and luteinizing hormone (LH) indicate that the output of the hypothalamus and pituitary is not being turned down as it would if the testes were responding normally to these hormonal signals. High levels commonly are considered an indication of a problem in the testes.

The Testicles, Epididymis,
and Vas Deferens

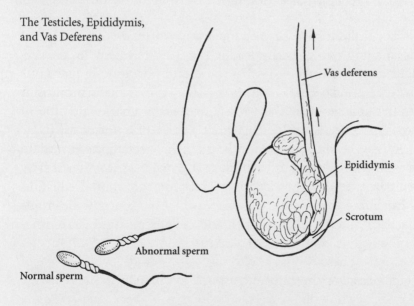

Vas deferens

Epididymis

Scrotum

Abnormal sperm

Normal sperm

The male and female reproductive systems work similarly in many ways: The hypothalamus pulses out GnRH, and that stimulates the pituitary to produce FSH and LH. These last two circulate in the bloodstream and help regulate the functioning of the ovaries and testes. In men, they stimulate the Sertoli and Leydig cells in the testes.

When stimulated by LH, the Leydig cells secrete testosterone, the hormone needed for bone and muscle growth, sexual development, and sperm production. To receive LH, Leydig cells need to have fully developed LH receptors, and the formation of such receptors requires FSH.

FSH also acts on the Sertoli cells that line the tiny tubes in the testes. Sertoli cells house the developing sperm cells in deep recesses, nurturing each sperm as it grows. And it's thought that FSH is necessary to help the testes themselves mature.

Treating Hormonal Problems

Although there have been many anecdotal reports of hormonal therapy improving sperm production, long-term studies that include control groups show that significant hormone-induced improvement in sperm levels is not sustained over many months. A positive change in several consecutive sperm tests in a period of weeks often leads to the belief that a particular hormonal treatment is successful. Sperm numbers can vary greatly from week to week, however, and studies that follow patients long term have demonstrated that such improvements often are short-lived.

Hormone treatments are expensive and can produce side effects such as aggressive behavior and weight gain, so if your physician suggests hormone treatment, you should ask further questions. These drugs should not be used routinely just because a man has a low sperm count, especially when hormone levels are normal. If your blood tests show that your hormone levels are normal, yet your doctor is recommending hormone treatments, you probably would be wise to avoid such therapy or to get another opinion.

We'd like to note, however, that there are a couple of disorders that may respond to treatment with hormones. These include instances in which FSH or LH levels are low because there's an abnormality in pituitary function, and in cases of hypogonadotropic hypogonadism (a rare genetic disorder), in which there's a chronic deficiency of the gonad-stimulating hormones.

Reduced FSH and LH Levels

Slightly lower-than-normal levels of FSH and LH may be the result of a problem in pituitary function that can't be diagnosed because it's too subtle. For some men, a regimen of 12.5 to 50 mg per day of clomiphene citrate may improve the release of FSH and LH and subsequent sperm production. (Clomiphene is a synthetic hormone that, in women, stimulates ovulation.) Semen analyses are performed about every three months to monitor sperm health and motility during this treatment.

The side effects of oral clomiphene therapy are mild and infrequent. They include breast enlargement, nausea, mild weight gain, dizziness, visual problems, and skin allergies, all of which will gradually disappear after the drug is no longer taken.

More severe deficiencies of FSH and LH can be treated with clomiphene in pill form or injections of one of the human menopausal gonadotropins available for treating infertility. If taken two or three times a week for three to six months, these drugs may return sperm production to normal levels.

Hypogonadotropic Hypogonadism

This is a rare gonad-deficiency disorder that occurs in fewer than one percent of infertile men, and it can be treated successfully with hormones. It's usually the result of the inadequate secretion of GnRH by the hypothalamus or a lack of FSH and LH secretion by the pituitary. Without the stimulation of these hormones, testicles are small and don't produce sperm. A man with this disorder also may have enlarged breasts and sometimes may lack a sense of smell.

This condition can occur before birth or afterward, sometimes as the result of an uncommon and usually benign pituitary tumor (adenoma) that affects that gland's ability to secrete the necessary levels of FSH and LH. Other reasons for this disorder include a damaged pituitary or a negative reaction to the use of anabolic steroids. If the cause is an adenoma, a diagnosis is made from measuring hormone levels in the blood, doing imaging studies, and finding defects in the person's visual fields that are caused when a pituitary tumor crowds the nearby optic nerve. Treatment may include removing the tumor if necessary, giving radiation therapy, replacing the missing hormones, or using a combination of these.

Genetic Disorders

A number of different genetic disorders can lead to inadequate GnRH production by the hypothalamus. Most common of these rare disorders is Kallmann's syndrome, which also may be accompanied by a very small penis, a decreased sense of smell, and undescended testicles. Another sign of Kallmann's syndrome is a delay in puberty and underdeveloped secondary sexual characteristics.

Overactive Pituitary or Underactive Thyroid

If your pituitary is overactive, the result often can be hyperprolactinemia, an excessive production of prolactin, which may cause breast enlargement, the inability to have an erection, and infertility. Other causes of high prolactin levels include liver disease, hypothyroidism, and the use of tricyclic antidepressants or certain antihypertension medicines.

Men with hyperprolactinemia also should undergo CT or MRI scans to check for a possible pituitary tumor, which can prompt the pituitary to overproduce prolactin as well as underproduce FSH and LH. Treatment for hyperprolactinemia is based on what's causing it. If the cause is an underactive thyroid, treatment with thyroxine, a thyroid hormone, often restores prolactin levels and fertility to normal. A large pituitary adenoma should be removed, even though these growths are usually noncancerous. A large adenoma not only can affect your fertility, it can also give you headaches, cause a type of diabetes, and, if it presses on your optic nerve, it eventually may damage your vision.

If medications are the cause of your hyperprolactinemia, they should be discontinued or replaced, if possible, with those that don't affect the pituitary. If the tumor is a microadenoma (which means it's small and benign) or if the cause of the high levels of prolactin can't be found, medical treatment in the form of bromocriptine may be used. Side effects of this drug can include low blood pressure, nausea, and vomiting. To reduce these risks, bromocriptine is given in very small doses.

IMMUNOLOGIC INFERTILITY

This is an uncommon condition that's difficult to diagnose and treat. In general, as a cause of infertility it's considered chiefly after other possible causes have been ruled out. It's theorized that the sperm of some men trigger an immune reaction against themselves, causing the production of antisperm antibodies (ASA). These antibodies cling to all parts of the sperm, hindering their ability to move through cervical mucus and to penetrate an egg cell. If large numbers of sperm are affected—over 80 percent—infertility may result.

Since sperm are generated long after birth, a protective mechanism appears to defend them from the body's usual automatic immune response to any protein material it wasn't born with. It's thought that sometimes this protective system breaks down, allowing sperm to be attacked by antisperm antibodies. Although not firmly identified as direct causes of such a breakdown, inflammation of the testicles, cancer, undescended testicles, varicocele, testicular trauma, biopsy, and vasectomy have been associated with the presence of ASA on sperm.

Diagnosis and Treatment

Both the diagnosis and treatment of this disorder are controversial and uncertain. When semen analyses reveal sperm that clump together rather than move separately, or sperm that don't move well by themselves, ASA-mediated infertility is viewed as a possibility— but only after all other reasons for infertility have been eliminated. Researchers list the following as indicators of possible immunologic infertility: (1) the existence of any of the medical events mentioned here, (2) a poor cervical mucus penetration test, (3) semen analyses that reveal sperm clumping together instead of moving separately, and (4) sperm that move weakly or not at all.

A number of methods for testing sperm for ASA are available, but accuracy can vary from lab to lab. Before treatment is undertaken, the results should be interpreted and verified by an experienced male infertility specialist.

Only men whose reproductive systems have no physical obstruction, whose partners have been studied fully, and who have the indicators just listed should be considered candidates for treatment. In general, only men whose ASA tests show that more than 50 percent of their sperm are antibody-bound usually are treated; sperm with fewer antibodies produce postcoital tests similar to nonaffected sperm.

Corticosteroid therapy is a common form of treatment that decreases antibody production and weakens antibody bonds. The results are not reliable, however. More than a dozen research studies using various dose levels of steroids produced pregnancy rates that ranged from 6 to 50 percent for the treated groups.

Intrauterine insemination (IUI) has been used to overcome the problem of poor sperm motility and the inability of ASA-bound sperm to penetrate the cervical mucus. Although much more expensive, this therapy is less risky than steroid treatment. However, studies using IUI as an answer to immunologic infertility have had small numbers of participants and their success rates were low and very variable. You'll find detailed information on IUI in Step 6A, pages 161–164.

Assisted Reproduction

The assisted reproductive technologies of IVF (in vitro fertilization), ZIFT (zygote intrafallopian transfer), and GIFT (gamete intrafallopian transfer) also have been used with moderate success to overcome male factor immunologic infertility. IVF and ZIFT have the advantage in demonstrating (before an egg is transferred to the uterus or a fallopian tube) whether or not it's been fertilized by the man's ASA-loaded sperm. These methods are discussed in the chapter "Extra Steps."

The results of many of these assisted reproductive technologies may depend on the percentage of sperm that's bound with ASA. In studies using IVF, pregnancy rates were higher among those couples in which fewer than 80 percent of the sperm were burdened with ASA.

The outlook is brighter today for couples who are having difficulty becoming pregnant because of male factor infertility. In just the last ten years alone, new technologies such as ICSI and a better understanding of the genetics of reproduction are making it easier to have babies despite obstacles that once seemed insurmountable. And we expect that the next decade will see the arrival of even more treatments to circumvent infertility.

QUESTIONS TO ASK YOUR DOCTOR

- ✎ If I should have male factor infertility, what treatments do you offer for this?

- ✎ Who performs these procedures?

- ✎ How often do they do them?

- ✎ If a live birth is considered a successful result, what is your success rate for the procedures?

- ✎ If my semen test is normal and my partner's tests have all been normal, would it make sense for me to have another semen test, just in case the first one was read wrong?

- ✎ If I had a sexually transmitted disease when I was younger, could it affect me now?

Extra Steps:
Choose Assisted Reproductive Technologies

Getting sperm and egg to meet and bond is not always simple. Because so many elements—such as overall health and weight, hormone levels, the timing of the reproductive system's complex chemistry, genetics, and the woman's age—are involved in conception, it's easy to understand why some couples may have great difficulty in getting pregnant. To assist couples to conceive whose reproductive systems are not working perfectly, medical science has devised a number of technologies that can bypass some of these obstacles. These assisted reproductive technologies, or ARTs, include in vitro fertilization (IVF), gamete intrafallopian transfer (GIFT), zygote intrafallopian transfer (ZIFT), freezing embryos, intracytoplasmic sperm injection (ICSI), and using donated eggs.

Such high-tech assists are just one part of a menu of fertility enhancements that may also include weight gain or loss, less exercise, stress reduction, ovarian stimulation, intrauterine insemination, and so on, from which you can choose those that are right for you as a couple. Your choices are likely to be affected by how you feel about each one, how much time you have, your religious beliefs, how much you can afford to spend, or what your health insurance will cover.

Moving along in a timely fashion is especially relevant if an assisted reproductive technology could be one of your choices. ART procedures are most successful when more than one healthy embryo develops, and such embryos can come only from healthy eggs. The ability to ovulate good eggs is closely related to your age, which means, if you're over thirty-five, you may not want to postpone ART. After age forty, it's not only more difficult to produce the necessary multiple eggs per cycle but also, as the eggs themselves get older, they're more likely to contain chromosomal defects. The embryos that develop from such eggs may be too imperfect to implant successfully or to develop into a healthy fetus.

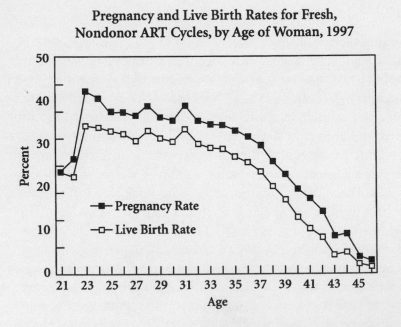

Pregnancy and Live Birth Rates for Fresh, Nondonor ART Cycles, by Age of Woman, 1997

A woman's age is the most important factor affecting the chances of a live birth when the woman's own eggs are used. This figure shows both the pregnancy and live birth rates for women of a given age who had an ART procedure in 1997. Both rates are relatively high for women in their twenties, but begin to decline among women in their thirties and older.

On the other hand, because ART is expensive and requires difficult physical procedures, it's good sense to try less costly and less invasive techniques first—if your tubes are not blocked, sperm health is not a factor, and you're closer to age thirty than to age forty. If time is on your side, you may get pregnant as readily with a change in lifestyle, a mind/body intervention program, or medication, as with an ART procedure. Nevertheless, you want to be careful not to stick with one type of treatment for too many cycles. A rule of thumb that we and many reproductive specialists recommend is to stay with a particular treatment for three to six cycles. Three cycles is the preferred length of treatment for many women. A discussion with your fertility specialist about moving to another procedure should include a consideration of the female partner's age and reproductive health, the quality of the male partner's sperm, and what you can afford.

As far as assisted reproductive technologies are concerned, the data is clear: the fourth, fifth, and sixth cycles have a decent pregnancy rate, but after three cycles, you are likely to feel that you're ready for a break, and you may wonder about continuing. This can be a good time to take a breather and consider once again how far you want to go with assisted reproduction and how attractive the alternatives may be.

SALLY'S STORY

We tried everything to conceive, including two IVF cycles, and nothing worked, although there was no medical reason for our infertility.

When the failures began to get to me and I felt infertility had taken over my life, I found Ali Domar's class. One of the things that particularly reached me was her saying that "if you really want to be a mother, you can. There is adoption." And then a nurse we knew told me of a reputable adoption agency that had healthy babies of Caucasian background. If we adopted, I didn't want a baby who was obviously not ours. I just didn't want us to look different as a family. At that time I had so many other issues to resolve about adoption I felt I couldn't deal with telling people our baby was adopted. My husband thought adoption was fine—he'd always said that if we wanted a large family we should have two of our own and adopt the rest. But I wanted a baby of my own.

We eventually called the agency and filled out its forms, although I still wasn't sure I wanted to adopt. And it was months before we actually started the agency's process of getting educated about adoption, thinking through issues we'd never considered, seeing the social worker, and all that.

We each had to write a letter to a prospective birth mother about ourselves, how we lived, how we would raise a child, what family meant to us, what we would tell the child about the birth mother. We sent them in, but I still didn't really believe this would happen—I'd heard so many stories about how difficult it was to find a baby. We were shocked when we received a telephone call almost immediately. A young woman had picked out our letters and thought we were the ones who should adopt her baby! We were stunned. We'd done nothing to prepare, and he was going to be ready for us in five days!

When we picked him up—the adoption became final twenty-one days after he was born, to give his mother a chance to change her mind—we were given all his birth records and the medical backgrounds of his parents and grandparents.

My husband bonded with our son the minute he picked him up in his arms, but it was the next day before I truly realized I was responsible for him, that I was now his mother. Today I can't imagine having a child I could love more. We feel he was meant for us, and we will probably adopt another child. All of this has made me realize that having a biological child may be all well and good, but what we really wanted was to be a family.

ART PROCEDURES

In 1978 the first baby conceived with the help of in vitro fertilization was born in England. Since then more than 100,000 couples have become parents either via IVF or the newer technologies (chiefly GIFT, ZIFT, and ICSI) that have grown out of IVF. In 1996, the last year for which we have data, 20,659 babies were born as a result of 64,036 assisted reproductive technology cycles. The majority were conceived with the help of IVF.

In Vitro Fertilization (IVF)

If you choose IVF, which is the assisted reproductive technology most frequently used today, you will be given a drug—a GnRH agonist—that will temporarily turn off your pituitary's secretion of the hormones FSH and LH, which ordinarily would cause your follicles to grow. One GnRH agonist, leuprolide, is given as a series of low-dose shots. Two drugs that have recently become available, Ganirelix and Cetrorelix, are given in one or two injections. Then, later in your cycle, precisely when they can be most effective in stimulating your follicles, you will be given FSH and LH by injection.

This technique, called down regulation, allows more control over the process of stimulating your ovaries and increases and controls follicle stimulation so that many enlarge at the same time. The result is the development of multiple follicles and eggs instead of the usual one. When it's time to retrieve eggs for the procedure, your doctor should be able to find mature eggs in the majority of the follicles.

As the follicles enlarge, they can be observed easily by ultrasound. In addition, your hormone levels will be monitored by blood tests. When an ultrasound shows that the follicles have become large enough to release mature eggs, you'll be given an injection of hCG to start ovulation. Because hCG usually causes eggs to start being released about thirty-six hours later, the procedure to retrieve them will be scheduled to take place just before they ovulate so that the eggs can be collected when they are most mature but before they leave the follicles.

Egg retrieval usually is performed as an outpatient procedure, even though an anesthetic is given, usually intravenously. When you are anesthetized, your eggs are removed from the ovary transvaginally—that is, via a long, hypodermic-type needle that reaches the ovary by being inserted through the top of your vagina. Using ultrasound as a guide, your physician will insert the needle into each mature follicle and use suction to gently draw out the egg and the fluid that surrounds it. The needle aspiration procedure takes twenty to thirty minutes. Afterward you will need an hour or two to recover, chiefly from the immediate effects of the anesthetic, before you feel able to go home. For a couple of days more, however, you can expect to feel tired and a bit hungover from the anesthetic.

Immediately after they're collected, eggs are fertilized in the laboratory by mixing them with your partner's sperm in a shallow petri dish or, if ICSI is being used, by injecting each egg with your partner's sperm. The fertilized eggs are kept warm and observed to see if they divide, beginning the process of becoming embryos, a stage that takes one to three days.

If the fertilized egg cells are dividing properly, after three days they've each become a four- to eight-cell embryo. The next step is to transfer the healthiest of these to your uterus, a process that doesn't require an anesthetic. (The health of an embryo is determined by examining it under a microscope to see how many cells it has—the more the better—and how symmetrical it is.) Your doctor will place a speculum in your vagina, clean your cervical area, and then slip the end of a catheter into your cervix. The catheter will contain fluid and the embryos. Using a syringe, this embryo/fluid mix is gently flushed into your uterus. This procedure is painless; it's much like having a Pap smear. Afterward you will have to remain lying down for thirty to sixty minutes. You also should plan to rest at home for at least twenty-four hours and not engage in strenuous exercise or intercourse for one to two weeks.

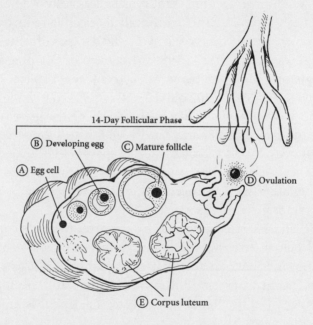

Ovary with follicles and eggs in various stages of maturity. After ovulating, an empty follicle becomes a cystlike corpus luteum and secretes progesterone.

The average number of eggs removed from an ovary is ten (depending on the woman's age); of the ten eggs, usually six will become fertilized in the lab and begin embryo development. If a woman is under age thirty-five, typically two embryos are transferred to her uterus; if she's older, two or three embryos are transferred. Both the couple and the woman's reproductive physician play a major role in deciding how many embryos should be moved to the uterus since there is always a chance that all the embryos will implant and grow into babies. At the same time, there is also a chance that none might implant. Whether embryos implant and develop normally depends on the quality of the embryos.

Although the pregnancy and birth of twins usually present few problems, triplets can produce more health challenges during pregnancy. If three or more embryos successfully implant, the couple may be offered a procedure called selective reduction, removing one or more embryos to avoid the dangers of a high multiple pregnancy and birth. In 1996, 61 percent of IVF pregnancies were singletons, 31.8 were twins, 6.5 percent were triplets, and 0.6 percent were quadruplets or quintuplets.

For the past ten years the live birthrate of IVF has increased at a fairly steady 1 to 2 percent a year. In 1996 it was 26 percent per treatment cycle; by the end of 2002, it's expected to be over 34 percent for each cycle that uses a woman's own nonfrozen embryos. These rates are based on procedures in which more than one embryo was transferred to the uterus.

As IVF success rates continue to improve, it has become increasingly clear that this method is most successful when the woman's ovaries have an adequate supply of egg follicles and the man has normal semen. Both the number and health of a woman's eggs decline after her teen years; the decline is more precipitous after age thirty.

Age is not the sole predictor of the health of your egg supply, however. The day 3 FSH test and the clomiphene challenge test, which are discussed more fully in Step 5, pages 135–136, are more definitive because they reveal whether or not the ovaries of an individual still respond to follicle-stimulating hormone. High levels of FSH on your cycle day 3 or after you have taken clomiphene for five days indicate that your ovaries are not responding normally, prompting the pituitary to pump out even more hormone. Studies show a close association between cycle day 3 FSH concentrations and IVF birthrates: high levels of FSH are linked to poor IVF outcomes.

Many couples have more than one factor contributing to their infertility and, in general, the more factors that are involved the less their chance of success with IVF will be. For instance, in one study of the impact of IVF on infertile women with endometriosis, the live birthrate per cycle was 31 percent for women whose only infertility factor was the endometriosis. If they had a male partner with an abnormal semen analysis, however, the live birthrate per cycle was 16 percent. For women who had both endometriosis and tubal disease, the live birthrate per cycle was 8 percent. Another study, of women with tubal disease, also showed declines in IVF success rates when additional infertility factors were present.

Among women who become pregnant after treatment with IVF, approximately 20 percent will experience a miscarriage and up to 5 percent will have a tubal pregnancy. Infants born as a result of IVF have a slightly higher than average risk of congenital malformations.

Gamete Intrafallopian Transfer (GIFT)

In GIFT, the medication regimen is the same as for IVF, but the woman's eggs are collected via laparoscopy and immediately mixed with her partner's sperm. The mixture is not retained in the lab, however, to observe if fertilization occurs and the eggs are dividing normally. Instead, sperm and eggs are combined in a catheter and, during the same laparoscopy, are transferred back to the woman, into the open ends of one or both fallopian tubes.

GIFT laparoscopy is done on an outpatient basis and usually requires general anesthesia. Three tiny incisions are needed for the laparoscope and other instruments. If you choose this method, your abdomen is inflated with gas to separate the organs so that the surgeon has a clear view of the ovaries and fallopian tubes. Needle aspiration is used to draw the fluid and egg from each mature follicle. While you are still under anesthesia, your eggs are separated from the fluid and combined with your partner's prewashed sperm in a catheter. In the meantime, the surgeon makes certain that your fallopian tubes are open and healthy. Then the mixture of gametes is transferred into one or both fallopian tubes. The abdominal incisions are closed with a stitch or two and, after a few hours in the recovery room, you'll probably be ready to go home. Again, it's a good idea to take it easy and avoid exercise and other strenuous activities for a week or so. If your abdomen is sore or you have pain from any gas that remains in your body—it usually migrates up toward your shoulders—you'll want to check with your doctor about taking a pain reliever. In fact, you might ask him about pain relief before you leave the hospital or infertility center. In 1996 the live birthrate for GIFT was 29 percent per treatment cycle.

This variation of ART was designed during the early days of assisted reproduction, when IVF success rates were low. GIFT developers found they could increase the number of pregnancies somewhat by putting eggs and sperm into the more natural nurturing environment of the fallopian tube as soon as possible. Because IVF success rates have increased steadily, the success rates for both procedures today are very similar. However, GIFT is used much less often, largely because it requires surgery and general anesthesia, is more expensive than IVF, and is considered slightly more risky. As of 1996, just over 5 percent of ART procedures performed in the United States were GIFT.

Zygote Intrafallopian Transfer (ZIFT)

This technique also was developed when IVF success rates were still fairly low and scientists were looking for variations that might offer greater success. Today it's rarely performed. IVF pregnancy rates have improved steadily, and currently there's little difference in the success rates of the two procedures. Furthermore, ZIFT involves two separate surgeries with anesthesia, a considerable strain for any woman. Because two operations are needed, ZIFT can cost more than GIFT and IVF.

Like GIFT, ZIFT requires functioning fallopian tubes. Eggs are retrieved transvaginally during the first procedure, as in IVF, mixed with sperm, and monitored for twenty-four hours, just long enough to make certain fertilization occurs. During the laparoscopy the next day, which requires several small incisions, the zygotes (embryos) are placed in one or both fallopian tubes, reducing the time they spend in a laboratory culture. The surgeries themselves and the recovery time they require are similar to GIFT.

Preserving Embryos

If, on average, six eggs are fertilized and begin the process of becoming embryos, and only two or three are used for an assisted reproduction procedure, what happens to the embryos that aren't used? In the 1980s it was discovered that embryos could be frozen safely, and if thawed and transferred to the mother's uterus months later, a certain percentage would grow into healthy babies. We should note, however, that the percentage of frozen embryos that become live births is less than it is for nonfrozen embryos. Preserving embryos this way has become an important part of ART; nevertheless, the decision to do this is entirely left up to the parents. Some couples are comfortable with this arrangement; others are not. Embryos that aren't chosen to be preserved are discarded or used for research purposes, according to the couple's wishes; poor-quality embryos are discarded.

Giving Sperm a Boost

Although ART procedures don't need large numbers of sperm, relatively speaking, and ART overcomes many of the hazards sperm face while trying to reach an egg, a minimum number (about 300,000 to 500,000) of active sperm still are necessary for success. Until recently, if a man's sperm were few in number, if they weren't very mobile or were unable to penetrate an egg, successful fertilization was unlikely. Today, however, ICSI, or intracytoplasmic sperm injection, is making genetic fatherhood possible for men who have little or no sperm in their ejaculate or sperm that aren't able to penetrate an egg. ICSI is described in detail in Step 6B, pages 184–187.

Donor Eggs

Assisted reproduction also makes it possible for a woman to donate her eggs to another woman who can't produce her own. Using standard IVF procedures, the eggs can be retrieved from the donor and fertilized in the lab with the prospective father's sperm, and the resulting embryos are transferred to the uterus of the intended mother. A uterus doesn't age at the same rate as ovaries and eggs, and quite often a woman can carry a pregnancy to term when it originates from eggs donated by a young woman. For the woman who has no eggs of her own, donor eggs usually are the only way she can become pregnant.

The probability of an embryo performing normally is strongly related to the age of the woman who produced the egg, rather than to the age of the recipient. The live birthrate for each ART cycle using embryos from donor eggs is in the 40 percent range, even for recipients who are over age forty.

Using an egg from a donor requires that the reproductive cycles of both donor and recipient be coordinated so that the recipient's uterus is ready for an embryo at the time egg retrieval from the donor occurs. For the recipient, hormone treatment can adequately stimulate her endometrium to prepare it for the arrival of two or three embryos and a successful pregnancy. Although this form of assisted reproduction is becoming more common, donor egg transfers are performed chiefly at larger fertility centers. Because eggs are not stored, making arrangements for a donor egg can take a number of months or more, depending on the source you use.

Couples may find egg donors through friends, relatives, fertility centers, and by advertising. There are about two hundred private egg donation agencies and clinics in the United States today, many of which have substantial information about their large number of potential donors. It's possible to use the Internet to peruse photographs of donors and their highly detailed backgrounds, which include information on their health, education, ambitions, and interests. Donors and recipient families can be matched right down to athletic talents, SAT scores, hair texture, and ability to tan. However, many clinics have waiting lists of people who want to use anonymous donors.

Because eggs cannot yet be frozen easily and subsequently tested for disease as sperm can, using fresh eggs—regardless of their source—raises the issue of disease transmission. However, such a risk is considered to be very small.

Clinic Success Rates—What Do They Mean?

Assisted reproductive technology has been used in this country since 1981 to help couples achieve a pregnancy, usually through in vitro fertilization. This treatment option is time-consuming and expensive, and making a decision to choose it can be very hard.

If you want to use ART and you're not already receiving infertility treatment at a center that offers these technologies, your next questions probably will be: How do I find a clinic and how do I get the basic facts about it, including its success rate? And even if you're already receiving treatment at an ART center, you might want to see how it compares to others in the area in its success with ART procedures.

Under federal law, the Centers for Disease Control and Prevention (CDC), in collaboration with the Society for Assisted Reproductive Technology and RESOLVE, a national consumer organization that helps infertile women and men, must publish the annual pregnancy and live birthrates of U.S. fertility clinics. The accuracy of the data that each clinic submits is verified by its medical director. Clinics and doctors that did not provide information also are listed.

Each one-page clinic report includes the characteristics of its program, the types of ART offered, and a summary of the diagnoses of the patients treated. Most important, of course, is the clinic's pregnancy and live birthrates, which are tabulated according to the woman's age: under thirty-five, thirty-five to thirty-nine, and over age thirty-nine. The success rates are summarized by the type of cycle: cycles using fresh embryos from nondonor eggs, cycles using frozen embryos from nondonor eggs, and cycles using donor eggs. Clinic information is listed in the report state by state. Because the data is based on live births, it takes at least nine months for the clinics to know their results. This information then is collected, tabulated, reviewed, and published. Thus, the clinics' 1996 experience with assisted reproductive technologies wasn't fully known until late 1997 and was published in 1998.

The report is called *Assisted Reproductive Technology Success Rates;* telephone the CDC at 770-488-5372 to receive the most recent one. You also can obtain ART information on-line through RESOLVE's Web page: www.resolve.org. If you want to ask on-line for the national report, on the RESOLVE Web page look for the CDC address: www.cdc.gov/nccdphy/drh/art97/index.htm. The Web page also offers other information, including a sampling of RESOLVE fact sheets on infertility, adoption, and related subjects.

The CDC notes that the size of an infertility program—the number of cycles it treats annually and the diagnoses of its patients—may affect its success rates. In general, the more cycles a center treats, the more skilled its staff becomes.

Four different measurements are used to depict ART success rates: *the pregnancy rate per cycle, the live birthrate per cycle, the live birthrate per egg retrieval,* and the *live birthrate per embryo transfer.* The *live birthrate per cycle* is the best measure to use when you are comparing the success of fertility centers.

The *pregnancy rate* is higher than the live birthrate because some pregnancies are lost through miscarriage, therapeutic abortion, and, in some instances, because of a stillbirth.

The *live birthrate* simply means the percentage of live births per ART cycle.

The *live birthrate per egg retrieval* generally is higher because it excludes cycles that were cancelled—that is, stopped before eggs were retrieved. Cycles are cancelled when too few egg follicles develop after the ovaries have been stimulated. Sometimes illness leads to a cancellation. In general, cycles are cancelled when the chance of success is poor because there were only one or two eggs.

The *rate of live births per embryo transfer* includes only those cycles in which an embryo or egg and sperm were transferred back to the woman. It excludes cycles in which no transfer occurred because the egg was not fertilized or the embryos that were formed were abnormal. As a result, this rate generally is higher than the rate of live births per egg retrieval.

The data supplied by the CDC is an excellent starting point for finding an ART clinic that achieves good results, but you may also want to ask other infertile couples who have used ART about their experiences. Support groups and RESOLVE may have useful information about fertility centers as well and often can be very helpful in facilitating the sharing of personal experiences. In addition, you will want to have your own interviews with the staffs of the clinics you are considering.

Clinics can show higher percentages of live births if they screen their candidates and take on as patients chiefly those who are likely to have good outcomes. Before you choose a clinic, you need to know what their entry criteria are: Do they accept patients of all ages; if not, what is the cutoff age? Do they accept women who have high cycle day 3 FSH levels? Or couples whose infertility may be caused by male factor problems? The criteria not only will let you know whether you might be accepted, but what's more important, it may explain why an individual fertility center has higher success rates than others in the area. More stringent criteria produce better results; however, such criteria and results may not always reflect the quality of a program. Sometimes a fertility center may look good on paper, but in practice it may not be the better clinic or the clinic that suits you best.

You will also need to know what a clinic's criteria are for cancelling a treatment cycle. If the policy is to cancel treatment because a patient hasn't produced what the clinic considers enough eggs, you may not wish to select it as your fertility center.

Furthermore, ask about the number of embryos the clinic routinely transfers to the uterus and what its rate of multiple births is. This information is included in the individual clinic fact sheet in the CDC report, but since the data in the report is at least three years old by the time it's published, you may want to see the clinic's current figures as well.

Using assisted reproduction can be an emotional, uncomfortable, and expensive process and it's important that you're at ease with the persons who'll be taking care of you. Doing some research and preparing your questions before you telephone or visit will help you be a more analytical consumer. Try to visit as many clinics as you can and don't hesitate to visit a clinic more than once. And don't be afraid to ask about every aspect of the procedures—the more you know the more at ease you'll be with the technology. The information you're gathering will help you make a good decision.

Trying to conceive is often apt to seem like one of the most difficult things you've ever done. Hopefully, this book has shown you that there are many approaches you can take. A lot of resources exist today to help you: skilled doctors, nurses, psychologists, social workers, support groups, organizations, and adoption resources. If you really want to be a parent, you can be—there *will* be a way.

QUESTIONS TO ASK YOUR DOCTOR

⤜ Do you specialize in infertility diagnosis and treatment?

⤜ Have you completed a fellowship in such diagnosis and treatment?

⤜ Do you have a subspecialty certification in reproductive endocrinology and infertility?

⤜ Which procedures do you (or your fertility clinic) offer? Do you perform ICSI?

⤜ Is a live birth your measure of success with these technologies? What is your per cycle live birthrate?

⤜ Do you have a statement showing your success rates?

⤜ Does your clinic provide emotional support services for the persons who are undergoing these treatments?

⤜ Do your patients have to meet certain criteria? What are they?

⤜ Do you cancel treatment cycles? For what reasons?

⤜ How many embryos do you usually choose to transfer to the uterus?

⤜ What do you do with embryos that are not used?

⤜ What is your rate of twins, triplets, and higher multiple births for the past three years?

⤜ Do you have a donor egg program for women who no longer can ovulate their own eggs?

Glossary

Acrosome reaction: the chemical change that enables a sperm to penetrate an egg.

Adenoma: a tumor that is usually noncancerous.

Adhesions: bands of inflammatory or scar tissue that join adjacent organs.

Andrology: the medical specialty that treats diseases of the male sex, particularly infertility and sexual dysfunction.

Anencephaly: the absence at birth of the brain, and the top of the skull. Most affected infants die within a few hours.

Antibody: a protein substance produced by the body in response to a stimulating substance.

Artificial insemination: a procedure that involves placing semen into the cervix by means of an instrument, instead of through sexual intercourse; see donor insemination.

Asherman's syndrome: a condition in which scar tissue formed in the uterus interferes with normal development of the uterine lining. May occur after a D&C.

Assisted reproductive technologies (ART): term used to identify procedures such as IVF, GIFT, and ZIFT.

Atherosclerosis: disease in which the inner layer of artery wall thickens, narrows the artery, and impairs blood flow.

Azoospermia: the absence of living sperm in the semen; the lack of sperm development.

Basal body temperature chart (BBT): a daily record of the body's temperature while at rest. After ovulation occurs, the temperature will rise 0.6 to 0.8 of a degree Fahrenheit.

Bicornuate uterus: a uterus with two separate cavities, each with its own fallopian tube.

Biopsy: removal of a fragment of tissue for study under a microscope.

Body mass index (BMI): a person's weight (in pounds) multiplied by 703, then divided by her/his height (in inches) squared.

Catheter: a flexible, fine tube used for aspirating or injecting fluids.

Catheterization: introduction of a catheter into a blood vessel, the uterus, bladder, or other organ.

Centrifugation: use of centrifugal force to separate substances of different densities.

Cervical mucus: mucus produced by the cervix that undergoes complex changes in its physical properties in response to changing hormone levels during the reproductive cycle. These changes assist the survival and transport of sperm.

Cervix: the lower part and neck of the uterus, an inch or so in length and less than an inch in diameter. It links the uterus with the vagina.

Chlamydia: a very common sexually transmitted infection that can cause internal inflammation and infertility.

Chorion: the outermost membrane enclosing a fetus; part of the placenta.

Chromosome: threadlike structures in a cell that carry the genes.

Cilia: hairlike projections in the fallopian tubes that move the egg or embryo toward the uterus.

Congenital conditions: certain mental or physical traits, malformations, or diseases that are present at birth; either hereditary or due to some occurrence during gestation.

Corpus luteum: a cyst formed in the ovary at the site of a ruptured follicle right after ovulation. It produces estrogen and progesterone during the second half of the ovulatory cycle.

Cryptorchidism: failure of the testicles to descend into the scrotum.

Culture medium: a liquid solution used to grow cells or tissue in a dish or test tube (in vitro) in the laboratory.

Day 3 FSH test: a blood test to measure the amount of FSH in the blood on day 3 of the ovulatory cycle. An unusually high amount of FSH is an indicator of unresponsive ovaries.

Diabetes mellitus: a disorder in which the pancreas produces insufficient or no insulin, causing abnormally high glucose levels in the blood. It leads to an accelerated degeneration of small blood vessels.

Diethylstilbestrol (DES): a synthetic estrogen thought to prevent miscarriage. It can cause abnormalities in the cervix, uterus, and vagina of the fetus.

Dilation and curettage (D&C): enlargement of the cervix in order to scrape or suction out the contents of the uterus.

Dominant follicle: the largest follicle on an ovary and the one in which an egg matures and ovulates.

Donor embryo: an embryo, usually frozen, and usually donated by a formerly infertile couple for whom IVF worked but provided too many embryos. The embryos are often donated to women unable to conceive with their own eggs. The donors relinquish all parental rights.

Donor insemination: insemination with sperm from someone other than the woman's partner; once termed artificial insemination.

Down regulation: the use of a hormone to stop the action of the pituitary gland and the ovaries.

Ectopic pregnancy: a pregnancy in which a fertilized egg implants outside the uterus, usually in the fallopian tube, ovary, or abdominal cavity. A dangerous condition that must receive prompt treatment.

Egg aspiration: removal of eggs from follicles during an IVF procedure.

Egg donation: an egg donated to a woman who cannot ovulate her own.

Egg retrieval: a procedure to collect the eggs contained in the ovarian follicles.

Ejaculate: the fluid or semen that carries the sperm out of a man's reproductive tract.

Ejaculatory duct: the tubes that carry sperm from the testicles to the urethra in the penis.

Embryo: an egg that has been fertilized by a sperm and undergone one or more cellular divisions.

Embryo cryopreservation: the freezing of healthy embryos that remain after IVF for possible future use.

Embryo transfer: placement of embryos into a woman's uterus via the cervix after in vitro fertilization or, in the case of zygote intrafallopian transfer, into her fallopian tubes.

Endocrinologist: a physician who specializes in diagnosing and treating problems regarding hormones or endocrine gland abnormalities.

Endometrial biopsy: removal of a sample of cells from the endometrium, the lining of the uterus, for study under a microscope.

Endometriosis: the presence of tissue similar to the lining of the uterus in other parts of the pelvic cavity.

Endometrium: the tissue lining the uterus that responds to estrogen and progesterone stimulation.

Epididymis: tightly coiled tubes that lead from each testicle, in which sperm are stored and matured for several weeks.

Erectile dysfunction: the inability to reach or maintain an erection long enough for intercourse; impotence.

Estradiol: the most potent form of estrogen released by the dominant follicle during ovulation.

Estrogen: a class of female hormones produced mainly by the ovaries from puberty to menopause.

Fallopian tube: one of a pair of tubes that conduct the egg from the ovary to the uterus. Fertilization normally occurs within this structure.

Fecundity: the ability to conceive.

Fecundity rate: the ability of a woman to conceive during any given month that ovulation occurs. Usually described as a percentage.

Fertile-type mucus: cervical mucus secreted around the time of ovulation that is distinctively abundant, slippery, and stretchy.

Fertilization: penetration of the egg by the sperm and the resulting combination of genetic material that develops into an embryo.

Fibroids: a common, benign muscle tumor of the uterus, often without symptoms.

Fimbria: fingerlike projections at the far end of the fallopian tubes that help collect the egg after ovulation.

Fimbrioplasty: the surgical procedure used to reconstruct tubal damage involving the distal (far) end of a fallopian tube.

Folate: the natural, but less absorbable form of folic acid.

Folic acid: the synthetic counterpart of folate that is absorbed about twice as efficiently as folate. Necessary to a woman's diet to reduce the risk of the birth defect of spina bifida.

Follicle: a small fluid-filled sac in the ovaries that nurtures a ripening egg. It secretes estrogen until the egg is ovulated, when it becomes the corpus luteum and starts to produce progesterone.

Follicle-stimulating hormone (FSH): a hormone secreted by the pituitary that stimulates follicle growth in the female and sperm production in the male.

Gamete intrafallopian transfer (GIFT): an ART procedure in which sperm and egg are placed in a fallopian tube via laparoscopy.

Gametes: the reproductive cells, either a sperm or an egg.

Genital warts: soft warts that grow in and around the vagina, the anus, and on the penis. They are transmitted by sexual contact, may lead to cervical cancer, and need prompt treatment.

Germ cells: the precursor of other cells—that is, the spermatid is the precursor cell of the sperm cell.

Gonadotropin: any hormone that stimulates the gonads (testes and ovaries).

Gonadotropin-releasing hormone (GnRH): the hormone released by the hypothalamus that prompts the pituitary to secrete other hormones (FSH and LH) needed for reproduction.

Gonads: the glands that produce the male and female gametes (sperm and eggs).

Gonorrhea: a sexually transmitted disease caused by the bacteria *Neisseria gonorrhoeae*. If the infection in women is not treated, it can spread to the cervix and fallopian tubes and inflame and damage them. In men, it can cause epididymitis and affect sperm quality.

Gram: a measure of mass and weight; one gram equals 0.035 ounce; one ounce equals 28.3495 grams (avoirdupois).

Hatching: the breaking out of the embryo from its outer membrane, the zona pellucida, in order to implant in the endometrium.

Herpes simplex: a sexually transmitted disease that produces a painful rash on the genitals. It cannot be cured. If a pregnant woman has an attack when the baby is due, a cesarean is performed to prevent infant infection during delivery.

Human chorionic gonadotropin (hCG): a hormone produced by the placenta; it can be injected to stimulate the ovaries to release an egg.

Human menopausal gonadotropin (hMG): a hormone extracted from the urine of postmenopausal women and used to stimulate both the testes and ovaries.

Hydrosalpinx: a fluid-filled sac formed in a fallopian tube when its far end is abnormally closed, causing fluid to accumulate.

Hypogonadotropic hypogonadism: a hormone deficiency that prevents sperm or egg production.

Hypospadias: a congenital defect in the penis in which the opening occurs underneath rather than at the tip.

Hypothalamus: a small area deep in the brain near the pituitary; it produces GnRH and other hormones that stimulate the pituitary.

Hypothyroidism: a condition caused by deficient production of thyroid hormone.

Hysterosalpingogram (HSG): an X-ray study of the female reproductive tract in which dye is injected into the uterus while X rays are taken to show the shape of the uterus and the degree of openness of the fallopian tubes.

Hysteroscopy: direct visualization of the uterus in order to evaluate any abnormalities that may exist. Most often this is done by inserting a hysteroscope into the uterus via the cervix.

Idiopathic: of unknown origin.

Implantation: the process by which the fertilized egg becomes attached to the lining (endometrium) of the uterus.

Impotence: the inability to achieve or maintain an erection long enough for intercourse. Also known as erectile dysfunction.

Infertility: the inability of a couple to conceive after twelve months of intercourse without contraception.

Interstitial: that portion of the fallopian tube that goes through the muscular wall of the uterus and opens into the cavity.

Intracytoplasmic sperm injection (ICSI): a procedure in which a single sperm is injected directly into a single egg.

Intrauterine insemination (IUI): an artificial insemination technique in which sperm are deposited directly in the uterus.

In vitro: literally "in glass," pertaining to a biological process or reaction taking place in an artificial environment, usually in a test tube or petri dish in a laboratory.

In vitro fertilization (IVF): the process of removing multiple eggs from the ovaries, fertilizing them in a petri dish in the laboratory, and transferring the resulting embryos into the woman's uterus.

In vivo: literally "in the living," referring to a biological process taking place in a living cell or an organism.

Kallmann's syndrome: a genetic disorder in men in which the hypothalamus fails to produce GnRH, resulting in FSH and LH deficiencies and lack of sperm production.

Klinefelter's syndrome: a male chromosomal and developmental disorder resulting in female characteristics and male sterility due to a lack of sperm production.

Laparoscopy: direct visualization of the ovaries, fallopian tubes, and uterus by means of a laparoscope, a long, narrow, illuminated instrument that enters the body through a very small surgical incision. Surgical procedures also may be performed using this method.

Laparotomy: surgery in which an incision is made through the abdominal wall, larger than that used in laparoscopy, to allow the visualization of reproductive structures for evaluation or surgery.

Leydig cells: the cells in the testicles that manufacture testosterone.

LH surge: the pituitary release of a large amount of LH to trigger the discharge of the mature egg from the follicle. It occurs about thirty-six hours before ovulation.

Luteal phase: the second half of the menstrual cycle, beginning with ovulation. Characterized by elevated levels of estrogen and progesterone.

Luteal phase defect: failure of the endometrium to develop in a timely fashion after ovulation, preventing implantation. This condition can be corrected with progesterone.

Luteinizing hormone (LH): a gonadotropin that, along with FSH, stimulates and directs the hormone and gamete production of the testes and ovaries.

Menstruation: the cyclical shedding of the lining of the uterus.

Microgram (mcg): one-millionth of a gram.

Microsurgery: surgery in which magnification and tiny instruments are used.

Milligram (mg): one-thousandth of a gram.

Miscarriage: loss of a pregnancy before the twentieth week.

Motility: the power of spontaneous movement.

Multifetal pregnancy reduction: a procedure used to decrease the number of fetuses a woman carries and improve the chances that the remaining fetuses will survive and develop into healthy infants.

Myomectomy: the surgical removal of fibroids (myoma) from the uterus.

Myometrium: the muscular outside wall of the uterus.

Needle aspiration: use of a fine needle to withdraw a bit of tissue for biopsy or an egg from a follicle.

Nucleus: the part of the cell that contains the chromosomes.

Occlusion: the state of being closed.

Oligospermia: scarcity of sperm in the semen.

Oocyte: another term for egg.

Ovarian dysgenesis: lack of eggs in the ovaries caused by a congenital condition.

Ovarian failure: a condition in which the ovaries do not contain follicles and eggs or do not respond to FSH stimulation.

Ovarian monitoring: using ultrasound and/or blood or urine tests to monitor ovarian follicle development and hormone production.

Ovarian stimulation: the use of drugs to stimulate the ovaries to develop follicles and eggs.

Ovaries: the two female sex glands that produce sex hormones and in which eggs develop; female gonads.

Ovulation: the release of an egg from the follicle.

Ovulation induction: the stimulation of follicle growth and egg release through the use of fertility drugs.

Pelvic cavity: the lower part of the abdomen that houses the uterus, fallopian tubes, and ovaries.

Pelvic inflammatory disease (PID): an inflammatory infection of the female reproductive organs, usually caused by a sexually transmitted disease.

Penis: the male sexual organ.

Petri dish: a shallow glass or plastic dish in which embryos develop during IVF procedures.

Pituitary adenoma: a benign growth in the pituitary gland that causes it to overproduce certain hormones.

Pituitary gland: a small gland at the base of the brain that secretes a number of hormones related to fertility.

Pituitary macroadenoma: a benign growth in the pituitary gland that is larger than 10 mm in diameter.

Placenta: a spongy, disc-shaped organ within the uterus from which the fetus derives its nourishment.

Polycystic ovarian syndrome (PCOS): the presence of irregular menstruation and excessive hairiness due to the development of many ovarian cysts, caused by an imbalance of hormones in the ovary.

Postcoital test: a test to determine whether the sperm/mucus interaction is normal—that is, whether sperm can move normally through the cervical mucus.

Premenstrual syndrome (PMS): the occurrence of all or some of the following symptoms in the week before menstrual flow: pain low in the back and abdomen, nervous irritability, headache, breast tenderness.

Progesterone: a steroid hormone secreted by the corpus luteum, which is formed in the ovary after ovulation. It is also the hormone that is responsible for maintaining early pregnancy.

Prolactin: a hormone secreted by the pituitary that stimulates breast milk production and supports gonadal function.

Prostaglandin: a hormone produced by the endometrium that causes the uterus to contract; one of a family of hormones that act in many tissues of the body.

Prostate gland: the male gland that supplies part of the fluid of the semen.

Proximal tubal blockage: an obstruction of the fallopian tube where it joins the uterus.

Puberty: the point in human maturation when sexual maturity occurs.

Receptor: the site on a cell to which a hormone attaches to express its function.

Retrograde ejaculation: a condition in which semen flows backward into the bladder instead of being ejaculated through the penis.

Salpingitis: inflammation of the fallopian tubes, sometimes caused by pelvic inflammatory disease.

Salpingostomy: a surgical attempt to re-create a normal fallopian opening and functioning fimbria in cases of a complete closing of the far end of the fallopian tubes.

Scrotum: the saclike structure that holds the testes.

Seminal fluid: the liquid that carries the sperm out of the male reproductive tract.

Seminiferous tubules: tiny ducts within the testes that are necessary for sperm production.

Septate uterus: a uterus divided by a fibrous wall.

Septic abortion: an infection that, on rare occasions, may occur after an abortion.

Sertoli cells: the cells within the testes that are involved in sperm cell production.

Sexually transmitted diseases (STDs): highly infectious diseases transmitted primarily by sexual contact, including syphilis, gonorrhea, chlamydia, herpes, and acquired immunodeficiency syndrome (AIDS).

Sperm: male reproductive cell.

Sperm motility: the ability of a sperm to move normally.

Sperm washing: diluting a semen sample with various tissue culture media in order to separate viable sperm from other components of semen.

Spina bifida: congenital defect in which part of the spinal column is missing; it allows the spinal membranes and sometimes the spinal cord to protrude.

Spontaneous abortion: miscarriage.

Sterilization: artificial blocking of the reproductive tubes of the male or female to prevent conception.

Syringe: a device used to inject or withdraw fluids.

Testicle: see testis.

Testis: also known as a testicle, the male sex gland in which sperm and testosterone are produced.

Testosterone: a male steroid hormone, or androgen, produced in the testes that affects sperm production and male sex characteristics.

Transvaginally: reaching into the lower abdomen with a long needle by going through the top of the vagina.

Tubal pregnancy: see ectopic pregnancy.

Turner's syndrome: a genetic abnormality in which the female is missing a chromosome and has no ovarian function.

Ultrasound: a noninvasive technique for visualizing a developing fetus and evaluating the development of the ovarian follicles.

Urethra: the duct leading from the bladder that conveys urine to the outside of the body.

Uterus: the muscular organ with a cavity lined with a layer of cells called the endometrium; its function is to nurture and protect the embryo/fetus.

Vagina: the channel in the female that connects the external sex organs with the cervix and uterus.

Varicocele: an abnormal twisting or dilation of the vein that carries blood from the testes back to the heart; a varicose vein of the testis. Occurs most often on the left testis.

Vas deferens: the duct that carries sperm from the epididymis to the posterior urethra.

Vasectomy: a surgically created obstruction of the vas deferens; used as a method of male sterilization.

Vasovasostomy: surgery to reverse a vasectomy.

Zona pellucida: the outer protein covering of the egg that the sperm first contacts during fertilization.

Zygote: a fertilized egg.

Zygote intrafallopian transfer (ZIFT): an ART procedure in which eggs are collected from the ovaries and fertilized outside the body. The resulting fertilized egg (zygote) is placed in a fallopian tube via laparoscopy.

Appendix

ORGANIZATIONS AND RESOURCES

Mind/Body Medicine (in general)

THE MIND/BODY MEDICAL INSTITUTE
Beth Israel Deaconess Medical Center
110 Francis Street, Suite 1A
Boston, MA 02215
617-632-9525

The tapes listed here can be ordered by writing to this address. Each tape is $10. No tax or postage is required. Please make checks payable to The Mind/Body Medical Institute, or MBMI.

✥ *Basic Relaxation Exercise/Mindfulness Meditation* (female voice). Side 1 (20 minutes) is a basic relaxation sequence to help elicit the relaxation response. Side 2 (20 minutes) teaches an awareness of sensation, thought, and sounds.

✥ *Basic Relaxation Response Exercise* (male voice). Side 1 (20 minutes) is similar to the preceding tape, plus it has breath awareness and body scan relaxation. Side 2 (45 minutes) has frequent pauses to allow you to practice techniques that elicit the relaxation response.

✥ *Advanced Relaxation Response Exercise* (female voice). Side 1 (30 minutes) guides you through a body scan relaxation, leading you into a relaxation response through awareness of your heart and repetition of your focus word. Side 2 (50 minutes) reinforces basic skills and also guides you through a stretching routine and a series of images for healing.

✤ *Guided Visualization with Ocean Sounds/Breath and Body Awareness* (female voice). Side 1 (24 minutes) is a body scan relaxation that incorporates guided visualization of a sandy ocean beach, with soothing ocean sounds in the background. Side 2 (30 minutes) leads you through a series of stretching exercises done in a sitting position to encourage a peaceful state of awareness and the relaxation response, without ocean background.

✤ *Relaxation Exercise/Mountain Stream Mental Imagery* (female voice). Side 1 (20 minutes) is a series of breathing techniques leading into body scan relaxation to alleviate tension from each body part and to practice breathing awareness. Side 2 (20 minutes) offers creative imagery during a walk through a forest to a mountain stream.

✤ *Extended Relaxation Exercise/Beach Walk Mental Imagery* (female voice). Side 1 (40 minutes) focuses on relaxation exercises, including a long body scan to relieve tension, then leads you through a visualization of a warm, comfortable bath. Particularly useful during medical, surgical, or dental procedures. Side 2 (20 minutes) guides you through breath and other exercises that elicit the relaxation response, followed by an imagery exercise of exploring a sandy beach on a magnificent day. (No wave sounds in the background.)

✤ *A Gift of Relaxation/Garden of Your Mind* (female voice). Side 1, Gift of Relaxation (20 minutes), introduces basic steps of eliciting relaxation response, plus deep breathing techniques to heighten your awareness and deepen your experience of the response. Side 2, Garden of Your Mind (20 minutes), includes body scan relaxation and breath awareness with imagery of a lovely garden.

✤ *Tuning In to Your Body, Tuning Up Your Mind* (female voice). Side 1 (30 minutes) guides you through chair and standing exercises that emphasize releasing physical tension, loosening joints, and realigning posture. It also encourages the elicitation of the relaxation response through mindfulness. Side 2 (30 minutes) offers instruction on floor exercises from *The Wellness Book* (see page 240), plus guidance for diaphragmatic breathing and using your breath to enhance your exercise. Diagram included.

↭ *An Introduction to the Relaxation Response/A Special Time for You* (female voice). Side 1 (20 minutes) introduces the practice of the relaxation response, diaphragmatic breathing, and release of physical tension. Good for someone learning the relaxation response. Side 2 (20 minutes) guides you through the relaxation response, using breath and nonjudging awareness to decrease tension and soothe physical discomfort.

↭ *Relaxation Exercises I and II* (female voice). Side 1 (20 minutes) includes a progressive muscle relaxation exercise. Side 2 (14 minutes) has nondistracting music that can be used for relaxation during exercise once the first side is no longer needed.

↭ *Relaxation Response Exercise Tape* (male voice). Side 1 (31 minutes) has instruction on eliciting the relaxation response during exercise. Side 2 (31 minutes) has nondistracting music for relaxation during exercise when the first side is no longer needed.

↭ *Basic Yoga Stretching Exercises/Stretching and Balancing Exercises* (female voice). Side 1 (20 minutes) is a series of gentle stretches and relaxation exercises to reinforce diaphragmatic breathing. Side 2 (20 minutes) is a slow-paced routine of stretching and movement awareness.

↭ *Rest in Gratitude/Healing Light* (female voice). Side 1 (19 minutes) uses guided imagery and soft music for a gentle body scan to achieve focused awareness and the relaxation response. Side 2 (19 minutes) uses breath awareness and ocean sounds to focus on a soothing, healing light for rest, healing, and deep relaxation.

↭ *Self-Empathy/Nurturing Change* (female voice). Side 1 (20 minutes) uses music and guided meditation to counter anxiety, plus breath focus to support nonjudging awareness, followed by body relaxation. Self-empathy, guided by self-awareness, is the focus. Side 2 (18 minutes) uses music and guided meditation to enhance self-awareness for greater physical and emotional well-being.

↭ *Positive Affirmations and Visualization in Weight Loss* (female voice). Side 1 (13 minutes), accompanied by soft music, uses affirmations to enhance positive thinking when you are dealing with food issues and body image. Side 2 (11 minutes) uses guided imagery that invites you into a gentle body scan. The tape ends with positive affirmations encouraging you to gain acceptance of where you are and who you are.

234   *Appendix*

❧ *Safe Place/Pain Visualization* (female voice). Side 1 (22 minutes) offers a guided meditation with progressive muscle relaxation and visualization of a safe place for patients with chronic pain. It is helpful for those who might experience anxiety or feelings of vulnerability during the relaxation response process. Side 2 (22 minutes) guides you through an advanced meditation with body sweeps of progressive relaxation and visualization of pain imagery. This can be a very helpful exercise for pain control.

❧ *Relaxation Exercises for Students—Tape 1* (female voice). Special Place/Worries in a Box/Music Relaxation 1 and 2/Mountain Meditation/Melting the Dime Spot (pain reduction).

❧ *Relaxation Exercises for Students—Tape 2* (male and female voices). Breath Focus Relaxation/Muscle Relaxation/Beach Walk/Garden Walk.

Mind/Body Medical Institute Affiliates

The Mind/Body Medical Institute has affiliates in several other states that offer programs for dealing with stress-related illness or illness complicated by stress, as well as instruction on relaxation and stress management. Some affiliates offer programs that deal specifically with the stress of infertility. For information on an affiliate in your area, contact Marilyn Wilcher, 617-632-9543. Or for a recent list of affiliates, check www.mindbody.harvard.edu.

In addition, Dr. Domar holds weekend infertility "retreats" for individuals and couples that compress the elements of the ten-session infertility program into two days. Retreats usually are offered twice a year in Boston or at other locations. For more information, call the main number of the Institute, 617-632-9530, and ask for Women's Health.

Organizations That Can Help

Endometriosis

ENDOMETRIOSIS ASSOCIATION
8585 North 76th Place
Milwaukee, WI 53223
414-355-2200

Infertility

RESOLVE
National Headquarters
1310 Broadway
Somerville, MA 02144-1779
617-623-0744
www.resolve.org

AMERICAN SOCIETY FOR REPRODUCTIVE MEDICINE
1209 Montgomery Highway
Birmingham, AL 35216-2809
205-978-5000
www.asrm.org

Offers listings of infertility support groups, surrogacy and egg donor programs, and mental health counselors and reproductive specialists by state, plus other information.

Mental Health

DEPRESSION AWARENESS, RECOGNITION AND
TREATMENT (D/ART) PROGRAM
National Institute of Mental Health
5600 Fisher's Lane, Room 15C-05
Rockville, MD 20857
301-443-4513

NATIONAL FOUNDATION FOR DEPRESSIVE ILLNESS
2 Pennsylvania Plaza
New York, NY 10121
800-248-4344

ANXIETY DISORDERS ASSOCIATION OF AMERICA
6000 Executive Blvd., Suite 513
Rockville, MD 20852-4004
301-231-9350

AMERICAN PSYCHOLOGICAL ASSOCIATION
750 First Street, NE
Washington, DC 20002
202-336-5500

Miscarriage

A.M.E.N.D.
4324 Berrywick Terrace
St. Louis, MO 63128
314-487-7528

SHARE
Pregnancy and Infant Loss Support, Inc.
St. Joseph's Health Center
300 First Capitol Drive
St. Charles, MO 63301
314-947-6164

Adoption

ADOPTIVE FAMILIES OF AMERICA, INC.
2309 Como Avenue
St. Paul, MN 55108
800-372-3300
www.adoptivefam.org

Offers information on adoption process, agencies, adoptive parent support groups, catalog of books and tapes that address multiethnic, independent, and international adoption issues. Adoptive Family Helpline available for answering questions.

NATIONAL COUNCIL FOR ADOPTION
1930 17th Street, NW
Washington, DC 20009-6207
202-328-1200/202-328-8072 (hot line)

An advocacy group that promotes national policies and high standards for adoption. Provides background information on adoption agencies, the name of the adoption licensing specialist in each state, and information on other adoption issues/problems.

NORTH AMERICAN COUNCIL ON ADOPTABLE CHILDREN
970 Raymond Avenue, Suite 106
St. Paul, MN 55114-1149
651-644-3036
www.nacac.org

Advocates chiefly for older children, sibling groups, multiethnic youngsters who are waiting for homes. Source of information on many issues, including international adoption and available subsidies for adopting children in foster care.

OPEN DOOR SOCIETY OF MASSACHUSETTS, INC.
1750 Washington Street
Holliston, MA 01746
800-93-ADOPT/508-429-4260

Most active in northeastern United States but has extensive lending library of books, tapes, and videos on all aspects of adoption accessible by mail. Holds monthly preadoption seminars and twice-yearly conferences for adoptive families and people thinking about adoption.

SOUTHEASTERN EXCHANGE OF THE UNITED STATES
P.O. Box 1453
Greenville, SC 29602
864-242-0460

Information source on adoption of older children, sibling groups, and children of different races.

Sources of Books on Health, Infertility, and Adoption Topics

OUR CHILD PRESS
P.O. Box 74
Wayne, PA 19087-0074
610-964-0606

PERSPECTIVES PRESS
P.O. Box 90318
Indianapolis, IN 46290-0318
317-872-3055

Nutrition Action Healthletter
THE CENTER FOR SCIENCE IN THE PUBLIC INTEREST
1875 Connecticut Avenue, NW, Suite 300
Washington, DC 20009-5728

SUGGESTED READING

American Yoga Association. *Easy Does It Yoga.* New York: Fireside/Simon & Schuster, 1999.

Benson, Herbert. *Timeless Healing.* New York: Scribner, 1996.

Benson, Herbert, and Miriam Klipper. *The Relaxation Response.* New York: Avon, 1976.

Benson, Herbert, Eileen Stuart, and the staff of The Mind/Body Medical Institute. *The Wellness Book: The Comprehensive Guide to Maintaining Health and Treating Stress-Related Illness.* New York: Fireside/Simon & Schuster, 1992.

Domar, Alice D., and Henry Dreher. *Self-Nurture: Learning to Care for Yourself as Effectively as You Care for Everyone Else.* New York: Viking, 2000.

Domar, Alice D., and Henry Dreher. *Healing Mind, Healthy Woman: Using the Mind-Body Connection to Manage Stress and Take Control of Your Life.* New York: Dell, 1997.

Lauersen, Niels, M.D., *Getting Pregnant: What Couples Need to Know Right Now,* rev. ed. New York: Fireside/Simon & Schuster, 1994.

Marrs, Richard, M.D., Lisa Friedman Bloch, and Kathy Kirtland Silverman. *Dr. Richard Marrs' Fertility Book.* New York: Dell, 1997.

Northrup, Christiane. *Women's Bodies, Women's Wisdom: Creating Physical and Emotional Health and Healing.* New York: Bantam, 1998.

O'Brien, Paddy. *Yoga for Women.* New York: HarperCollins, 1995.

Schiffmann, Erich. *Yoga: The Spirit and Practice of Moving into Stillness.* New York: Pocket Books, 1996.

Tobias, Maxine. *Complete Stretching Book.* New York: Random House, 1992.

Sources

Step 1: Begin Making Healthy Lifestyle Changes Today

"Avoiding the Fracture Zone." *Nutrition Action Healthletter.* April 1998.

Bolumar, F., et al. "Caffeine Intake and Delayed Conception: A European Multicenter Study on Infertility and Subfecundity." *American Journal of Epidemiology* 145, no. 4 (1997):324–34.

Clark, A. M., et al. "Weight Loss Results in Significant Improvement in Pregnancy and Ovulation Rates in Anovulatory Obese Women." *Human Reproduction* 10 (1995):2705–12.

Dlugosz, L., et al. "Maternal Caffeine Consumption and Spontaneous Abortion: A Prospective Cohort Study." *Epidemiology* 7 (1996):250–55.

Fenster, F., et al. "Caffeinated Beverages, Decaffeinated Coffee, and Spontaneous Abortion." *Epidemiology* 8 (1997):515–23.

"Folic Acid: For the Young and Heart," *Nutrition Action Healthletter.* September 1995.

Frisch, R. E. "Body Fat, Menarche, and Fertility." In the *Encyclopedia of Human Nutrition.* London: Academic Press, 1998.

———. Paper presented at the annual meeting of the American Association for the Advancement of Science, Boston, February 1988.

———. "Fatness and Fertility." *Scientific American,* March 1988:88–95.

Goldstein, M. "Of Babies and the Barren Man." *Scientific American,* Summer 1999:74–79.

Green, B. B., et al. "Risk of Ovulatory Infertility in Relation to Body Weight." *Fertility and Sterility* 50 (1988):721–26.

Grodstein, F., et al. "Self-Reported Use of Pharmaceuticals and Primary Ovulatory Infertility." *Epidemiology* 4 (1993):151–56.

Grodstein, F., M. B. Goldman, and D. W. Cramer. "Infertility in Women and Moderate Alcohol Use." *American Journal of Public Health* 84 (September 1994):1429–32.

Hadi, H. A., J. A. Hill, and R. A. Castillo. "Alcohol and Reproductive Function: A Review." *Obstetrics and Gynecology Survey* 42, no. 2 (1987):69–74.

Hakim, L. S., and R. D. Oates. "Nonsurgical Treatment of Male Infertility: Specific Therapy." In Larry I. Lipshultz and Stuart S. Howards, eds., *Infertility in the Male*, 3rd ed. St. Louis: Mosby, Harcourt Brace, 1996.

Hakim, R. B., R. H. Gray, and H. Zacur. "Alcohol and Caffeine Consumption and Decreased Fertility." *Fertility and Sterility* 70, no. 4 (October 1998): 632–37.

Jensen, T. K., et al. "Does Moderate Alcohol Consumption Affect Fertility? Follow-up Study Among Couples Planning First Pregnancy." *British Medical Journal* 37, no. 22 (1998):505–10.

Mahajan, A. K., et al. *Annals of Internal Medicine* 97, no. 2 (1982):357.

Netter A., et al. *Archives of Andrology* 7, no. 1 (1981):69.

"New Standards for Nutrients." *Harvard Women's Health Watch*. June 1998.

Ondrizek, R. R., et al. "An Alternative Medicine Study of Herbal Effects on the Penetration of Zona-Free Hamster Oocytes and the Integrity of Sperm DNA." *Fertility and Sterility* 71, no. 3 (1999):517–22.

Smith, E. M., et al. "Occupational Exposures and Risk of Female Infertility." *Journal of Occupational Medicine* 39 (1997):138–47.

Stanton, C. K., and R. H. Gray. "Effects of Caffeine Consumption on Delayed Conception." *American Journal of Epidemiology* 142, no. 12 (1995): 1322–29.

Tas, S., R. Lauwerys, and D. Lison. "Occupational Hazards for the Male Reproductive System." *Critical Reviews in Toxicology* 26, no. 2 (1996): 261–307.

"Vitamins and a Mineral: What to Take." *Nutrition Action Healthletter*. May 1998.

Windham, G. C., et al. "Moderate Maternal Alcohol Consumption and Risk of Spontaneous Abortion." *Epidemiology* 8 (1997):509–14.

Wynn, M., and A. Wynn. "Slimming and Fertility." *Modern Midwife* 4, no. 6 (June 1984):17–20.

Zhang Hua and K. R. Loughlin. "The Effect of Cocaine and Its Metabolites on Sertoli Cell Function." *Journal of Urology* 155 (1996):163–66.

Step 2: Maximize the Response of Your Reproductive System

Bar-Chama, N., and D. J. Lamb. "Evaluation of Sperm Function." *Urologic Clinics of North America* 21, no. 3 (1994):433–46.

Marrs, Richard, Lisa F. Bloch, and Kathy K. Silverman. *Dr. Richard Marrs' Fertility Book.* New York: Dell, 1997.

Step 4: Ease Emotional Stress

American Medical Association. *The Encyclopedia of Medicine.* New York: Random House, 1989.

Demyttenaere, K., et al. "Anxiety and Conception Rates in Donor Insemination." *Journal of Psychosomatic Obstetrics and Gynaecology* 8 (1988): 175–81.

Domar, A. D., and M. M. Seibel. "Emotional Aspects of Infertility." In Machelle M. Seibel, ed., *Infertility: A Comprehensive Text.* Norwalk, CT: Appleton & Lange, 1990.

Domar, A. D., et al. "The Prevalence and Predictability of Depression in Infertile Women." *Fertility and Sterility* 58, no. 6 (1992):1158–63.

Domar, A. D., P. C. Zuttermeister, and R. Friedman. "The Psychological Impact of Infertility: A Comparison with Patients with Other Medical Conditions." *Journal of Psychosomatic Obstetrics and Gynaecology* 14, (1993):45–52.

Domar, A. D., and H. Dreher. *Healing Mind, Healthy Woman: Using the Mind-Body Connection to Manage Stress and Take Control of Your Life.* New York: Dell, 1997.

Domar, A. D., R. Friedman, and P. C. Zuttermeister. "Distress and Conception in Infertile Women: A Complementary Approach." *Journal of the American Medical Women's Association* 54, no. 4 (1999).

Domar, A. D., et al. "Impact of Group Psychological Interventions on Pregnancy Rates in Infertile Women." *Fertility and Sterility* 73, no. 4 (2000):805–11.

Lapane, L. K., et al. "Is a History of Depressive Symptoms Associated with an Increased Risk of Infertility in Women?" *Psychosomatic Medicine* 57, (1995):509–513.

Thiering, P., et al. "Mood State as a Predictor of Treatment Outcome After In Vitro Fertilization/Embryo Transfer Technology." *Journal of Psychosomatic Research* 37 (1993):481–91.

Step 5: Take Advantage of Nature

Barbieri, R. L. "Infertility." In Samuel Yen, ed., *Reproductive Endocrinology.* Philadelphia: Saunders, 1999.

Collins, J. A. "Unexplained Infertility," In W. R. Keye, et al., eds., *Infertility: Evaluation and Treatment.* Philadelphia: Saunders, 1995.

Institute of Medicine. *Science and Babies.* Washington, DC: National Academy Press, 1990.

Rein, M. S., M. D. Hornstein, and R. L. Barbieri. "The Infertile Couple." *Kistner's Gynecology.* St. Louis: Mosby, Harcourt Brace,1999.

Step 6A: Find and Treat Anatomical Problems in the Woman

Barbieri, R. L. "Infertility." In Samuel Yen. ed., *Reproductive Endocrinology.* Philadelphia: Saunders, 1999.

"Better Safe Than Sorry." *Newsweek* Special Issue, March 1999:54–55.

Guzick, D. S., et al. "Efficacy of Superovulation and Intrauterine Insemination in the Treatment of Infertility." *New England Journal of Medicine* 340, no. 3 (January 21, 1999):177–83.

Harvard Medical School. "Health of Women." *Harvard Medical School Family Health Guide.* New York: Simon & Schuster, 1999.

Marrs, R., Lisa F. Bloch, and Kathy K. Silverman. *Dr. Richard Marrs' Fertility Book.* New York: Dell, 1997.

Step 6B: Diagnose and Treat Male Problems

Anderson, D. J. "The Effect of Genital Tract Infection and Inflammation on Male Infertility." In Larry I. Lipshultz and Stuart S. Howards, eds., *Infertility in the Male,* 3rd ed. St. Louis: Mosby, Harcourt Brace, 1996.

Berger, Gary S., M. Goldstein, and M. Fuerst. *The Couple's Guide to Fertility.* Garden City, NY: Doubleday, 1994.

Coburn, M., E. D. Kim, and T. M. Wheeler. "Testicular Biopsy in Male Infertility Evaluation." In Lipshultz and Howards, eds., *Infertility in the Male.*

Gilbaugh, J. H., III, and L. I. Lipshultz. "Nonsurgical Treatment of Male Infertility: An Update." *Urologic Clinics of North America* 21, no. 3 (1994): 531–48.

Goldstein, M. "Of Babies and the Barren Man." *Scientific American,* Summer 1999:74–79.

Harvard Medical School. "Health of Men." *Harvard Medical School Family Health Guide.* New York: Simon & Schuster, 1999.

Lahn, B., and K. Jagalian. "The Key to Masculinity." *Scientific American,* Summer 1999:20–25.

Laumann, E., A. Paik, and R. C. Rosen. "Sexual Dysfunction in the United States, Prevalence and Predictors." *Journal of the American Medical Association* 281, no. 6 (1999):537–44.

Nagler, H. M., R. K. Luntz, and F. G. Martinis. "Varicocele." In Lipshultz and Howards, eds., *Infertility in the Male.*

Page, D., S. Silber, and R. Oates. "AZFc Deletions Transmitted by ICSI." *Human Reproduction* 14, no. 7 (July 1999):1722–26.

Thompson, S. T. "Prevention of Male Infertility: An Update." *Urologic Clinics of North America* 21, no. 3 (1994):365–76.

Veldhuis, J. D. "Male Hypothalamic-Pituitary-Gonadal Axis." In Lipshultz and Howards, eds., *Infertility in the Male.*

Extra Steps

American Society for Reproductive Medicine. *ASRM Bulletin* 1, no. 6 (April 27, 1999).

Barbieri, R. L. "Assisted Reproduction." In Samuel Yen, ed., *Reproductive Endocrinology.* Philadelphia: Saunders, 1999.

Centers for Disease Control and Prevention. *1996 Assisted Reproductive Technology Success Rates, National Summary and Fertility Clinic Reports.* Washington, DC: U.S. Department of Health and Human Services, 1998.

Illustration Credits

Index

Harvard University, 83
Mind/Body Program for Infertility, 20, 86–94
Hatching, 54
Hatha yoga, 106–8
Headaches, 96
Herbal remedies, 40–41
Herpes simplex, 151
High blood pressure, medications for, 38, 180, 198
Hormonal irregularities, 130–32
alcohol and, 33
antidepressants and, 83, 132–33, 198
body fat and, 31, 33
cervix and, 161
male, 38, 194–99
smoking and, 37
stress and, 81, 83–84, 93
see also specific hormones
Hot water, avoiding, 42–43, 57, 180
Human chorionic gonadotropic (hCG), 54, 141–43, 207–8
Human menopausal gonadotropin (hMG), 142–43, 173
for male infertility, 197
side effects of, 143–44
Humegon, 142
Hydrosalpinx, 159
Hyperprolactinemia, 198–99
Hypogonadotropic hypogonadism, 197–98
Hypospadias, 190
Hypothalamus, 31, 46, 49, 50, 55, 194, 195
dysfunction of, 130–32, 197, 198
fertility drugs and, 139–40
stress and, 83
Hypothyroidism, 198–99
Hysterectomy, 168
Hysterosalpingography (HSG), 137, 153–54, 158, 165
Hysteroscopy, 157, 168, 169

Imagery, guided, 98–102
Imipramine, 194
Immune response
to embryo, 54
to sperm, 199–202
Implantation of embryo, 53–54, 60
Impotence, 178–80
atherosclerosis and, 37
drinking and, 35
medications causing, 39
stress and, 84
treatment of, 180–82
In vitro fertilization (IVF), 50, 118, 139, 147, 174, 184, 203, 207–12, 215
cost of, 79
depression and pregnancy rate from, 82
exercise and, 106
immunologic infertility and, 201
intracytoplasmic sperm injection and, 185
relaxation techniques before, 100
religious prohibitions on, 77–78
smoking and, 37
success rates for, 126
surgery versus, 157, 173
Infections, 58
after hysterosalpingography, 154
male infertility due to, 183
after miscarriage or abortion, 153
pelvic, fallopian tube problems from, 151–52
prompt treatment of, 41
Infertility, causes of, 128
Insulin, 133
Intercourse, 52
fertility drugs and, 140
frequency and timing of, 43–44, 176–77
Internet, 117, 124
Intracytoplasmic sperm injection (ICSI), 118, 184–87, 201, 203, 207, 208, 213–14

Asherman's syndrome after, 169
caffeine and, 36
fertility drugs and, 141
immunity factors in, 54
infection after, 153
after in vitro fertilization, 211
uterine abnormalities and, 166–68
Mood swings, 120, 141
Mucus, cervical, *see* Cervical mucus
Müllerian ducts, 164
Multiple pregnancies, 141, 143, 144,
    210
Multivitamin/mineral tablets, 26–28
Mumps, 183
Myomectomy, 168

Needs, attending to your own, 102–6
Negative thoughts, changing, 110–12
Neomycin, 39
Nicotine, 37–38
Nitrofurantoin, 39
No, learning to say, 115–17, 123
NoDoz, 36–37
Nurturing yourself, 102–6, 117
Nutrition, 22–28, 123
    poor, impotence and, 179

Obesity, 32–33
Obstetrician/gynecologists, 124
Oligospermia, 184, 185
Oocytes, 46, 134
Ovarian cancer, 146–47
Ovarian dysgenesis, 137
Ovarian failure, 134–35
    diagnosing, 135–36
Ovarian hyperstimulation, 144
Over-the-counter drugs, caffeine in,
    36–37
Ovulation, 45–48, 50–52, 128
    alcohol and, 33
    body mass index and, 32, 33
    cessation of, 84
    determining, 61–66

exercise and, 20, 31
impaired, 127, 130–37
intercourse during, 43–44, 59,
    176–77
test kits, 65–66
tests for, 129
thyroid replacement therapy and, 39
treatments for problems with, 118,
    137–49

Paired listening, 114–15
Pants, tight, 42, 180
Pap smear, 160
Papooseroot, 41
Parlodel, *see* Bromocriptine
Partner communication, 114–15, 123
Pelvic inflammatory disease, 123,
    151–52
Pelvic surgery, 151, 152
Penis
    abnormal opening of, 190
    in Kallman's syndrome, 198
Pesticides, 41
Phenylpropanolamine, 194
Pituitary gland, 39, 49, 50, 55, 194, 195
    dysfunction of, 130–32, 197–98
    fertility drugs and, 140, 145
    in vitro fertilization and, 207
    overactive, 198–99
    stress and, 83, 84
Placenta, 60
Pleasing yourself, 102–6, 123
Polycystic ovarian syndrome (PCOS),
    133, 143
    surgical treatment of, 147–48
Polyps, uterine, 157
Prayer, 96, 97
Prednisone, 141–42
Premature births, 144
    uterine abnormalities and, 165, 166,
    168
Premature ovarian failure, 134–36
Premenstrual syndrome (PMS), 84, 86